MW01292902

The Physical Therapy Advisor's Guide to

TREATING
LOW BACK PAIN
DURING EXERCISE AND ATHLETICS

*Complete with Prevention
and Rehabilitation Strategies*

Ben Shatto, PT, DPT, OCS, CSCS

Publishing services provided by

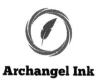

Archangel Ink

ISBN-10: 1548117102

ISBN-13: 978-1548117108

TREATING LOW BACK PAIN (LBP) DURING EXERCISE AND ATHLETICS VIDEO PACKAGE

To help guide you through **Treating Low Back Pain (LBP) during Exercise and Athletics,** I have created a package that you can get access to which includes a 7-part series of instructional videos in which I address the following:

- Low back pain prevention during exercise

- Specific warm ups for exercise and activities

- What really is the "core" and why it matters

- Treatment techniques (including how to apply Kinesiological tape)

- Long term management strategies

Don't miss out on this nearly 60 minutes of actionable advice to prevent and treat LBP as it relates to active individuals, sports, and athletics!

There is also an additional bonus eBook, **Preventing and Treating Overtraining Syndrome**, in which I show you how to recognize the risk factors and symptoms of Overtraining Syndrome (OTS). You'll learn how to utilize prevention strategies to help you develop a personal training strategy that will allow you to push past your limits and prior plateau points in order to reach a state of what is known as overreaching (your body's ability to "supercompensate"). This will speed up your results, so that you can train harder and more effectively than ever before! In addition, learn how to use the foam roller (complete with photos and detailed exercise descriptions) as part of a health optimization program, recovery program, rest day or treatment modality.

CONTENTS

AUTHOR'S NOTE

This rehabilitation guide has been written and categorized into very specific sections that target different aspects and time periods during a person's injury and recovery process. Although it's best to read this rehabilitation guide in sequential order, it can also be used as a reference guide for specific aspects of a lumbar injury or recovery. For example, you may initially only be interested in reading the **Low Back Pain (LBP) Prevention Strategies** while someone else may only be interested in **Initial Treatment**.

There are certain aspects of each section that may have repeated information because the rehabilitation guide is written in such a way that information can be independently read. I intentionally created the content this way in order to make it easier for those that will choose to read the sections out of sequence on a more as needed basis.

Throughout this rehabilitation guide, I reference books, exercise equipment, products, supplements, topical agents, and web sites that I personally use and recommend to my family, friends, clients, and patients (for use in the clinical setting). For your reference and convenience, please refer to the **Resource Guide**.

PREFACE

I had waited all year for the City of Trees half marathon. My goal (as always) was to post a PR (personal record) for the event. Since it was a fairly flat course, I figured it would be a good opportunity to run fast (at least, fast for me). As part of my training protocol, I was squatting two days per week and working on general leg strength and cross training (practicing yoga) one day per week.

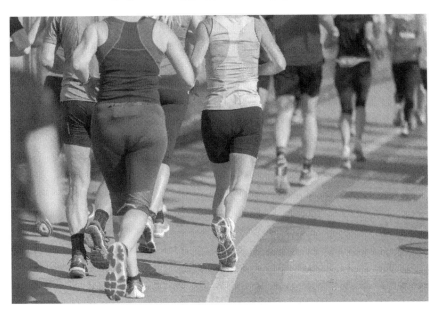

My back had been sore off and on for almost five years. Medical professionals didn't offer me any specific reasons as to why. Neither chiropractic nor physical therapy seemed to help much, so I just ignored it. But not this day!

I had just completed my second work set of squatting at the gym. At the time, I wasn't experiencing any notable back pain. I was on my second repetition and on my third set when my low back gave way. The weight came down and hit the rack safety rails! **My back hurt, but worse, it felt unstable.** I decided to leave the gym in shame. I picked up the weights I was using, but the pain began to worsen.

By the time I drove home, I could barely get out of my truck. I decided I was tough, so I took some ibuprofen and still went to work. By the time I made it to the office (about 10 minutes), I was in real trouble. I walked around for a while, and I took some Tylenol before I decided to go home. I got in my truck, but by then the pain was so bad that I couldn't push in the clutch or hardly use the brakes. I really don't know how I make it home that morning, but I needed help from my wife to get out of my truck.

It only got worse from there. I went to lie on my bed. Again, another bad plan! An hour later when I needed to urinate, I realized I couldn't even get out of bed! **The pain was worse than anything I had ever experienced.** After much struggle and help from my dad (who was called in to help), I was able to get upright, only to break out in a cold sweat, start shaking, and nearly pass out from the pain. Still having to urinate, I experienced one of the more humbling things I have ever done. I had to ask for help from my wife to urinate into a plastic bottle because I couldn't get out of bed.

Long story short, I went to a doctor who diagnosed me with low back pain (LBP) from a lumbar strain and prescribed pain medication and a steroid pack. After many more days of pain, I was finally upright again.

A month later, I was ready to start back into my training, but frankly, I was nervous! My back felt weak, and I had no idea how much was too much. The worst part of it all: I'm a physical therapist! Shouldn't I known what to do? It sure didn't feel like it at the time.

The medication did mostly relieve the pain, but I had a chronically sore back that felt weak and unstable. I was performing physical therapy exercises and stretches. I was even using heat and electrical muscle stimulation (EMS).

My treatment wasn't helping me that much. At least, not to the point that I felt I could get resume my training for my upcoming half marathon. **All I wanted to do was to get back to training, but I was too scared to!**

This experience started me down a path of study that changed my life. I realized how incompetent I had been as a physical therapist who treated others experiencing severe low back pain. I had new appreciation for those patients who wanted to get back to their sport and activity. I also realized that my prior physical therapy interventions were not preparing people to get back to sport nor most high level activities.

What do you do when you're past the worst of the pain and want to resume training, but you don't feel physically, mentally or

emotionally ready? Your insurance money may be used up. The pain may have dissipated, but you're still not sure how to progress through the next steps. What if it happens again? Can I train as hard as before? Am I really better? I have lost so many days of training, should I even compete in my event?

Often after a severe case of low back pain, you may be too scared to train like you did prior to the injury, and it turns out you should be! *At least until you understand why low back pain almost always re-occurs and what you can do to prevent it.*

INTRODUCTION

Did you know that an estimated $50 billion dollars is spent annually on back pain related issues? It affects nearly 80% of the U.S. population at one time or another. It's one of the top reasons for physician and physical therapy visits and one of the most common reasons for missed work days. **The best training plan in the world won't do us much good if we're unable to implement that plan due to pain and/or injury.**

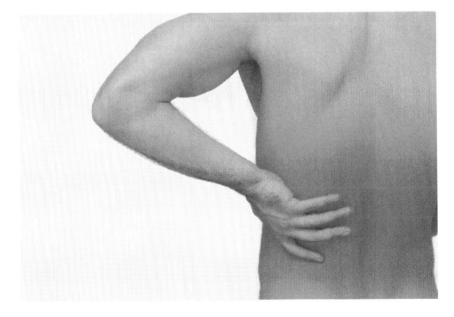

When reviewing research or anecdotal evidence online, there is no shortage of articles, blogs, and opinions regarding low back pain (LBP). But what about a specific resource for the athlete, the weightlifter, the CrossFitter or the runner who is experiencing low back pain during exercise? How does an athletic population know how to handle episodes of LBP? What specifically can an athlete or active person do to avoid low back pain to lessen the risk of injury and lost training days?

The prevention and rehabilitation strategies outlined in this rehabilitation guide answer those questions. **You will learn how to safely self-treat your low back pain and helpful methods for a speedy recovery.** (Not to mention, possibly saving you time and money by avoiding a physician visit!)

The good news is that participating in sports, running, CrossFit, and weightlifting doesn't increase your risk of developing LBP. On average, being in good health, physically fit, and active actually decreases your risk. Occupations involving heavy manual labor or bending over while working in a field don't appreciably increase your risk. However, there are specific behaviors to avoid when possible.

Eliminating your risk factors is a key step in avoiding low back pain and injury in general. The ideal goal is to execute a perfectly designed training plan for your sport or activity. In order to achieve this, you must remain healthy and be able to carry out the training plan. An injury can derail such plans if you don't properly address your known risk factors.

RISK FACTORS FOR LOW BACK PAIN (LBP)

Fortunately, most low back pain (LBP) is mechanical--meaning it is from a physical or structural cause and isn't typically related to more serious conditions such as cancer or infections. Structural pain is often caused from an injury to the disc, ligamentous tissue or the cartilage associated with the smaller facet joints that help make up the transvers processes of the spine. Although muscle related pain is often related to these types of injuries, it's typically due to muscle spasming as the muscle attempts to splint and stabilize the injured area. It's often diagnosed as a lumbar muscle sprain, but that is rarely the cause of the pain.

This rehabilitation guide is geared specifically for addressing mechanical LBP pain that can be specifically changed through specific movements either better or worse. *(All other forms of pain must be evaluated by a medical physician.)*

The problem with most mechanical LBP is not that it is serious, but that it is very painful and reoccurs. People who have had an episode of mechanical LBP are 90% more likely to experience it again. It's best to minimize your risk factors for experiencing LBP by being pro-active. Let's discuss many of the most common risk factors.

- **SMOKING.** Smoking is a major risk factor for LBP. The chemicals in cigarette smoke affect the lungs' ability to exchange oxygen and the body's normal healing response. These chemicals alter the blood supply to the discs and other spinal structures which affects nutrient exchange and increases the risk of pain. Healing time for all medical conditions worsen with smoking. Smoking significantly increases failure rates after back surgery.

- **GENDER.** Males have a higher risk of LBP. Females tend to experience more cervical or neck pain. (Obviously, you have very little control over this factor other than the knowledge that you're at an increased risk if you are a male.)

- **GENETIC PREDISPOSITION.** A family history of low back pain increases your risk. In some cases, this may be due to actual structural deformities which may be genetically linked. More commonly, it's a learned behavior, such as chronic sitting and slouching (poor posture or movement patterns), that can lead to a higher risk of LBP.

- **PRIOR EPISODES OF LBP.** Once you have experienced LBP, you are more likely to have re-current episodes. This is partially due to weakness in the deep multifidus muscles (*as shown on page 18*) that help to support the spine and prevent shearing forces on the spinal discs and ligaments. In the presence of pain or injury, the multifidus muscles reflexively stop functioning as well. They do not return to normal function without specific exercise training. This weakness can be addressed with proper physical therapy intervention. Improper timing of when the muscles contract before and during movement is also a factor when considering the muscles of the inner core.

- **PREGNANCY.** Pregnancy increases your risk for LBP due to structural changes as the baby develops as well as hormonal changes. The expectant mother releases relaxin, a hormone which loosens (relaxes) ligamentous tissue of the whole body (particularly, the pelvis) to prepare for the baby's delivery. Most women can manage the pain by modifying posture and movements while learning techniques for self-management of the pain (such as massage or the use of heat or ice). Specific braces to help stabilize the sacroiliac joint or to help support the weight of the stomach may also be helpful.

- **SEDENTARY LIFESTYLE.** A sedentary lifestyle will increase your risk for LBP. The spine is designed to work and move. In order for the spine to remain healthy, it requires exercise and movement.

- **PROLONGED SITTING.** Sitting for more than two hours a day not only affects your general health status in a negative way, but it also increases your risk for LBP. Sitting on a vibrating surface increases your risk further. Heavy equipment operators are likely to experience LBP as sitting is combined with vibration. Sitting in a chair is one of the most common reasons for why people suffer from LBP. In other cultures (where squatting is the norm and no one typically sits in a chair), episodes of LBP, knee pain, and hip pain are significantly less. Also interesting is that they are rarely constipated in comparison.

For runners, sitting is one of the biggest risk factors for developing LBP. This may seem odd, but many runners like to travel for destination races. The travel entails sitting when driving to the event and then afterward. This is especially bad if the return trip is right after the race (same day). Sitting (slouched in particular) causes excessive strain on the lumbar discs and ligaments. It also leads to tight hamstrings and hip flexors. It also generally tends to inhibit proper gluteal muscle (a known risk factor for piriformis pain). Now combine all of these risk factors with running 26.2 miles and a long car ride!

- **POOR POSTURE.** Typically this involves a slouched or forward flexed posture which causes your pelvis to posteriorly tilt and flatten your back. Work to maintain your normal lumbar curve when you stand and sit. In western culture, we spend most of our day sitting slouched or standing hunched over. This is an excellent way to increase your risk for LBP. Sitting with poor posture is one of the major risk factors for disc herniation and development of arthritis and spinal stenosis.

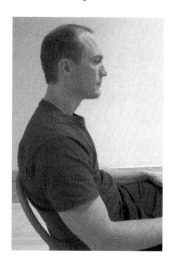

- **NO WARM UP PRIOR TO EXERCISE.** This is a common mistake which can lead to injury. Jump out of your bed in the morning without warming up, and then start your running or exercise routine. *(Please don't!)* Instead, prepare your body for challenging activities in order to avoid injury. Spinal discs are more vulnerable to injury the first 60 minutes of the day due to the prolonged immobility at night and an increase in size as they absorb interstitial fluid around them. This is why you are taller first thing in the morning. This is also why your spinal discs are more prone to injury immediately upon waking. A proper warm up (particularly, in the morning) is critical.

  A warm up should consist of a cardiovascular component, a thorough spinal warm up (more thoroughly discussed in **The Warm Up** section) and a dynamic stretching routine of the actual exercises you will be performing to insure that you're ready for the movement. This is pertinent for most activities including: weight-lifting, CrossFit, soccer, basketball, and running. A proper warm up is not only critical in the morning, but it's also in the afternoon or evening (particularly, if you have spent most of the day sitting or immobile).

- **CONTINUING TO EXERCISE EVEN WHEN EXHAUSTED.** This is a common problem among CrossFitters and/or when you're performing High Intensity Training (HIT). It can also be an issue on the long run days or if other factors are affecting you. Exhaustion has the potential to result in poor technique, which increases your risk that the body will not be able to handle the intensity of the exercise. It can result in injury, such as a muscle pull, tendon strain, joint injury or lumbar injury.

When performing HIT, hill repeats, and/or intervals, you must maintain proper form and technique. If you are unable to perform the exercise/activity with proper technique, then you need to either stop and rest or taper down the intensity. Poor technique will eventually lead to injury. Often during a long run, the back can become fatigued from the static posture or prolonged pounding of each step over time which can lead to injury. Try to avoid running on hard surfaces, such as concrete, which increases the strain and load on the spine. Continuing activity past the point of exhaustion increases your risk of injury.

- **POOR TECHNIQUE.** Poor technique, along with feeling exhausted, often occurs when performing exercises that are too advanced. Performing unfamiliar lifting techniques or lifting too much weight will likely result in poor technique. The most common issue in regard to poor technique is inadequate range of motion (ROM) to allow for a proper movement pattern to occur. This could be in a weightlifting technique, running or a sport specific activity. Your body requires adequate ROM to insure that a proper technique can even be performed.

If you cannot properly perform the technique, then you should not be performing the exercise with a high load, heavy weight or rapid pace. Keep the load lighter and improve your ROM. Take the time to learn the proper techniques. Please see your coach, athletic trainer or physical therapist for the proper technique for your activity of choice.

- **HIGH TRAINING VOLUME WITHOUT REST.** Who needs a rest day? All of us can benefit from taking a break.

Training every day without regard to rest is an excellent way to cause over training syndrome and injury. Tissues need adequate rest and recovery to properly function, grow, and develop.

- **POOR EQUIPMENT OR TRAINING ENVIRONMENTS.** Using poorly fitting equipment, such as wearing improper footwear or a too small or too big of a weight belt, also increases your risk of injury. Poor training environments, such as prolonged running on concrete (a hard surface), also lead to a greater strain on the joints of the body and in particular, the lumbar spine. Always use properly fitting equipment and train in the right environments.

Other risk factors, including certain medical conditions, can affect bone, muscles or the spine directly. Some risk factors are out of our control; many others can be addressed. *Be mindful of your risk factors and be pro-active in maintaining a healthy back!*

HOW TO PREVENT LOW BACK PAIN (LBP)

CORE MUSCLES

Often when we hear about low back pain, we also hear about the core muscles. Core muscles are part of the body's natural method of stabilizing the spine. The body uses many different techniques and systems to help support the spine during all of its movements and activities. The vertebrae themselves actually interlock through the facet joints for stability along with the lumbar discs. In addition, there are many ligaments that help to support the spine in all four directions. After you get past the boney stability and the ligamentous stability, the body uses the **core muscles** to provide muscular stability in combination with intra-abdominal pressure to form a round cylinder that is utilized to support the spine. This is accomplished using muscular support through the **core** musculature.

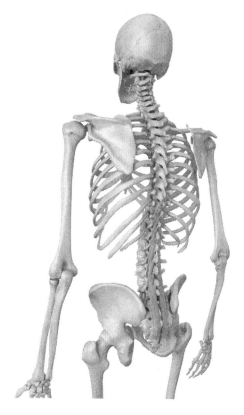

The Multifidus Muscles

The core actually consists of two separate groups of muscles. The **inner core** consists of the muscles of the pelvic floor, the transversus abdominis (TVA), diaphragm, and the multifidus muscles (shown above) that extend from vertebrae to vertebrae along the back side of the spine. The TVA wraps all the way around the stomach and attaches to the spine via a thick fibrous fascial layer known as the thoracolumbar fascia. This is what helps to form the cylinder. The cylinder is a more stable and solid structure. When the TVA is contracted in conjunction with the pelvic floor and diaphragm, there is an increase in the intra-abdominal pressure which is also helpful for spinal stability and support. When this is performed in conjunction with the outer core muscles, it's known as the Valsalva maneuver.

THE PELVIC BRACE

The pelvic brace refers to co-contraction of the pelvic floor muscles, the transverse abdominal muscles, and the multifidi. These muscles have such a strong role in stabilization. (This is not a Valsalva maneuver.) It's crucial to re-teach the trunk to stabilize itself because the associated stabilizing muscles have been known to shut off (not activate fully) after back injury. These muscles are hardwired to work as a team as they stabilize the spine. Once you can get one group activating correctly, it's much easier to get the others as well.

The important part of the stability that the pelvic brace offers is through motor control and timing. These muscles need to activate a split second prior to an exercise or activity. They would normally perform this without conscious thinking, but in cases of injury, the timing is off. The actions need to be performed manually until they are once again working correctly. This will vary and is dependent on your severity of your injury and associated pain. It generally takes 1-3 weeks to perform normally with intermittent ongoing practice.

In order to activate the pelvic brace, begin with locating the **pelvic floor**. For most people, this will be the easiest muscle group to activate. An easy way to locate the pelvic floor is to contract the muscles that stop the flow of urine or the muscles that keep you from passing gas. You can practice **Kegel** exercises. *If you suffer from urinary incontinence, performing Kegel exercises will have a signif-*

icant benefit for you and in many cases can eliminate incontinence almost entirely.

Sit on a chair with your feet and knees wide apart. Try to lift the muscles of your pelvic floor away from the chair. People sometimes accidentally contract the muscles of the buttocks and upper leg when learning to isolate the pelvic floor. Don't let it happen, and remember to keep breathing and relax. It is easy to try too hard on this exercise. Another cue that is sometimes helpful is to think about utilizing the muscles that would be necessary to stop urinating mid-flow or to stop you from passing gas.

STRENGTHENING THE PELVIC FLOOR

Once you have learned to isolate the pelvic floor muscles, you will begin strengthening them by holding the contraction and repeating it multiple times. **Research indicates that in order to rehabilitate the pelvic floor, a person should work up to 10 second holds performed 30-80 times per day (throughout the day). If you cannot contract the pelvic floor for 10 seconds, start at 3 seconds and work up.** Contract the pelvic floor as you breathe out. Just like weightlifters that exhale as they exert themselves, the muscles of the inner core should be contracted while exhaling and exerting.

Once you can perform the pelvic floor contraction, begin to work on strengthening the pelvic brace. You need to control the three parts of the inner core (pelvic brace): the pelvic floor, the transverse abdominals, and the multifidus.

The Pelvic Brace: Lie down with your knees bent, and take a belly (diaphragm) breath. Breathe out, and lift your pelvic floor muscles as you tighten your transverse abdominals and your multifidus. Avoid contracting your buttocks, thighs, or "six-pack" abdominal muscles. Avoid tilting your pelvis, and keep breathing. **Hold the pelvic brace for at least 3 seconds (your goal is 10 seconds), and repeat 30-80 times per day.**

Once you learn the pelvic brace, integrate it when sitting, and then into your daily activities. *The ultimate goal of pelvic bracing is to retrain your inner core, so that you will automatically pre-tense the muscles that protect your low back before performing potentially damaging activities such as lifting, pushing, and pulling.*

The second group of muscles that help to support your back are known as the **outer core muscles**. These muscles are responsible for movement of the trunk and spine as well as helping with stability. The inner core muscles do not actually help to produce any trunk or spine gross movement. The outer core muscles consist of a group of muscles known as the lumbar paraspinal muscles, the quadratus lumborm, the internal and external obliques, and the psoas major and minor. Some may want to add the quadriceps, glutes and hamstrings (basically, any muscle that attaches to the pelvis). That is okay, but I tend to place them in another category. Notice that the rectus abdominis ("the six pack" muscles) are not listed as it is responsible for lumbar flexion, but it doesn't add much in the way of spinal stability although they look cool!

Another common term that is utilized frequently when referring to spinal stability is the **posterior chain**. The muscles of the posterior chain are often defined as the lumbar paraspinal muscles (the muscles that extend the spine, the back extensor muscles), the glutes, and hamstrings. Although there is overlap in the definitions of the posterior chain and outer core muscles, I like to differentiate the two groups of muscles. Both are equally important. The posterior chain muscles work hand in hand with both the inner core and outer core muscles.

Weakness in the core muscles and posterior chain muscles is highly correlated with low back pain. Unfortunately, the muscles of the inner core become highly dysfunctional in the presence of spinal pain or injury. These muscles will reflexively shut down and decrease their activation. **This is one reason why once you have suffered an episode of low back pain, you are more likely to suffer from subsequent episodes.** This is also why it is critically important to prevent the first episode of low back pain. Thankfully, the treatment of choice in almost all cases involves exercise.

GENERAL PREVENTION
FOR LOW BACK PAIN (LBP)

Research for low back pain (LBP) prevention (particularly for athletes and fitness enthusiasts) is minimal. Most of the recommendations are similar to a sedentary population and primarily addresses posture and prolonged sitting. These general recommendations are accurate and helpful, and they should be incorporated into a prevention strategy. However, such basic recommendations don't fully address all of the needs for prevention for those of us who like to push ourselves in a particular sport or activity.

I have combined research with known anatomical and physiological principles in order to develop very specific strategies for general LBP prevention among athletes such as sport enthusiasts, CrossFitters, weightlifters, and runners. These principles are helpful for anyone participating in athletics as well as those implementing a healthy lifestyle. Throughout this rehabilitation guide, my intent is to address specific causes of LBP as well as the best practices on how to prevent and self-treat when you experience an episode of LBP.

- **IF YOU SMOKE, STOP.** Smoking is one of the top risk factors for developing LBP. Even cutting back can decrease your risk.

- **LIMIT YOUR SITTING.** Limit the amount of sitting that you spend at one time. Move from your sitting position every hour, and ideally, walk. If you aren't able to walk, then try to shift your position at least once every twenty minutes. Frequent position changes can help to avoid LBP. Avoid a long car trip directly before or after a long run or a race. For destination races and/or events, it's best to arrive at least a day or two early and wait a day prior to returning home.

- **SIT WITH CORRECT POSTURE.** Whenever possible, make sure that your knees stay below your hip level and that you are able to maintain your natural lumbar curve. A **McKenzie lumbar roll** is a great tool to help you maintain correct posture (*as shown on page 31*).

- **IMPLEMENT A WALKING ROUTINE.** Walking has many health benefits. It helps to improve circulation and blood flow into the spinal discs which allows for vital nutrient exchange. It provides a gentle range of motion to the spinal structures. Walking is also helpful for the following reasons: releases stress reducing hormones; releases hormones that can control blood sugar levels for up to 24 hours; burns calories; and helps to prevent constipation. Walking in a fasted state can help your body to learn how to utilize fat more efficiently as an energy source. It is also a weight bearing activity that can be beneficial in reducing osteoporosis.

Your walking routine should be a separate lifestyle habit apart from your typical exercise routine (which may or may not include walking). Your walking routine should be incorporated into your daily life as part of a healthy lifestyle. Since sitting is a risk factor for LBP, getting up and taking short frequent walking breaks is an excellent way to provide the necessary nutrients to your spine. If you would like more information regarding the general health benefits of walking, please visit: **www.ThePhysicalTherapyAdvisor.com** and refer to **Why Walking is Critical to Your Health** and **Why You Should Walk Not Run**.

- **EAT HEALTHY.** A healthy diet is critical to avoiding injury. Your tissues need nutrients to help them perform at a high level. Avoid process foods as much as possible, limit sugary food, and add more protein and healthy fat in your diet. Maintaining a diet with adequate healthy fats is essential in providing the nutrients to support all hormone function in the body as well as support the brain and nervous system. Adequate protein intake is necessary to support muscle health and development.

  Poor eating can lead to diabetes, which increases your risk of LBP. Diabetes also affects your body's ability to heal. If you experience an episode of LBP, it may be more difficult to recover from. Lumbar discs do not have a good blood supply. Diabetes, which is a microvascular disease, affects the small capillaries of the body. Smoking also decreases your body's ability to deliver vital nutrients to the spine and discs. Weight gain and obesity contribute to altered movement patterns. A lack of movement increases your risk of developing LBP.

- **HYDRATE.** The human body is primarily made of water, which is critical for all body functions. Adequate water intake is critical to avoid dehydration which can negatively affect your training as well as the function of the discs. Dehydrated tissues are prone to injury as they struggle to gain needed nutrients to heal and repair. Dehydrated tissues are less flexible and tend to accumulate waste products.

Stay hydrated by drinking water. Try to avoid beverages that contain artificial sweeteners or chemicals with names you can't spell or pronounce. If the beverage contains caffeine or chemicals that you cannot pronounce, then they do not count toward your daily water intake. Water, herbal teas, and coconut water are appropriate. Sports drinks, fitness waters with artificial sweeteners, and soda (diet or regular) may actually cause more harm and lead to dehydration.

Although this recommendation sounds simple, I find that very few of us are properly hydrating. This becomes even more important when there is an injury present. The goal is to remain hydrated throughout the day. Drinking smaller amounts more frequently can be more helpful than a large amount once or twice a day. You may need to increase your potassium, sodium or calcium intake to help you absorb the fluids. Sometimes drinking pure water or distilled water will simple flush out your system, but is not necessarily absorbed by your tissues.

You may also consider adding sea salt or a specific liquid mineral supplement. **Sherpa Pink Gourmet Himalayan Salt** contains the electrolytes you would expect as well as a host of other trace minerals. I have found that adding in sea salt can be highly effective when treating muscle cramps and soreness. I highly recommend it to anyone who is suffering from chronic cramping or after participating in an athletic event. *Drink a small glass of*

warm water, mixing in a teaspoon full of pink Himalayan sea salt.
Since it absorbs into your tissues better with the added salts, you are less likely to need to urinate overnight. Coconut water is also an excellent way to hydrate and provides added nutrients without the added calories. Be sure to skip the coconut water with artificial sweeteners.

- **SUPPLEMENT.** If you are training at a very high level or regularly engaged in high volume training, I like to add supplementation as part of an injury prevention strategy. I often will cycle my supplementation routine to go hand in hand with my training routine. As my training intensity and volume increase, I take additional supplements as part of my recovery and prevention protocol.

  I recommend a supplement known as **CapraFlex by Mt. Capra**. Essentially it combines an organic glucosamine and chondroitin supplement along with several other natural herbs designed to reduce inflammation.

  Another supplement called **Tissue Rejuvenator by Hammer Nutrition** also contains glucosamine and chondroitin as well as a host of herbs, spices, and enzymes to help support tissues and limit inflammation.

  I recommend taking either **CapraFlex** or **Tissue Rejuvenator**, but not both. I typically recommend that you try a 14-30 day protocol initially to see how your body responds. If you find it helpful, I recommend that you take 2/3 of a dose as part of a maintenance strategy or during high volume or over reaching portions of your training cycle.

Another supplement I occasionally recommend for those engaging in a very high level of training is a colostrum supplement called **CapraColostrum by Mt. Capra.** Colostrum is the first milk produced by female mammals after giving birth. It contains a host of immunoglobulins, anti-microbial peptides, and other growth factors. It is especially good at strengthening the intestinal lining which prevents and heals conditions associated with a leaky gut. Colostrum can also help a person more effectively exercise in hotter conditions. Over all, it can boost the immune system, assist with intestinal issues, and help the body to recover faster.

Please consult with your pharmacist and/or physician prior to starting any new supplementation protocol. Herbs could interact with some medications particularly if you are taking blood thinners.

LOW BACK PAIN (LBP) PREVENTION DURING EXERCISE

The following prevention strategies are designed to be best practice for avoiding episodes of low back pain (LBP). They should also be considered best practice for enhancing sport performance along with a specific recovery protocol. *Your recovery protocol should be as intentional and programmed as your actual training sessions and routines.*

These prevention strategies include specific details on what to do before, during, and after performing exercise or a competitive event.

SITTING

Sitting is a major risk factor for LBP. Sitting (slouched in particular) causes excessive strain on the lumbar discs and ligaments. It also leads to tight hamstrings and hip flexors. It generally tends to inhibit proper gluteal muscle function.

Now consider a lengthy car or plane ride when traveling to compete in a race or competition. Then combine prolonged sitting with running 26.2 miles or playing a soccer match or performing at a weightlifting competition.

The risk factors for travel are not just in going to the event, but the return travel can be equally risky, if not more. (Avoid traveling on the same day as the event.) Your body's tissues just performed a very taxing event. Sitting in a prolonged slouched posture doesn't allow for proper blood flow or nutrient exchange. The risk factors for injury just went up exponentially.

- **LIMIT YOUR SITTING.** Limit the amount of sitting that you spend at one time. Move from your sitting position every hour, and ideally, walk. If you aren't able to walk, then try to shift your position at least once every twenty minutes. Frequent position changes can help to avoid LBP. Avoid a long car trip directly before or after a long run or a race. For destination races, it's best to arrive at least a day or two early and wait a day prior to returning home. As soon as you arrive at your destination, perform the **Extension Biased Stretches for Low Back Pain** and **Leg and Pelvic Stretches for Low Back Pain** (as demonstrated in the **Rehabilitation Guide**). If you must travel back the same day, then you need to plan on very frequent stops to allow for walking and specific recovery stretches.

This advice on limiting sitting is not confined to runners traveling to the next race or weightlifters driving to the next competition. In general, sitting takes a cumulative effect on the spine. Sitting while at your office or on the couch for the past last several weeks and/or months adds up. Sitting all day at the office, then going to exercise without an adequate warm up is just as risky as sleeping all night, then performing an intense training session without an adequate warm up. As part of your prevention, implement a walking routine, sit less, and properly warm up prior to exercise to insure that your spine is ready for activity.

- **SIT WITH CORRECT POSTURE.** If you are going to sit, then make sure you have a proper sitting posture. Whenever possible, make sure that your knees stay below your hip level and that you are able to maintain your natural lumbar curve. A **McKenzie lumbar roll** is a great tool to help you maintain correct posture. It provides you with mechanical feedback to help maintain your normal curve. Below I demonstrate where to position the lumbar roll to help you to stop slouching.

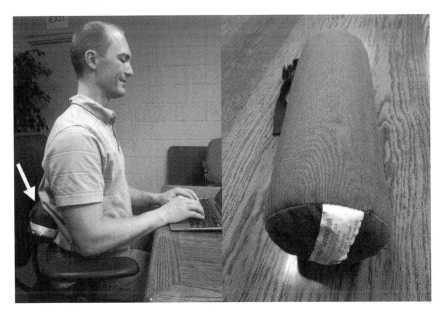

THE WARM UP

Unfortunately, the warm up is often marginalized. A common excuse for skipping the warm up is usually due to a lack of time. A thorough and specific warm up should never be skipped. *A proper warm up not only helps you limit your risk of injury, it will also allow to you train and perform at a higher more intense level.*

A proper warm up should be a multifaceted approach. The idea is to prepare the body for movement and activity. If the exercise or activity is to be performed first thing in the morning or after a day of sitting or sedentary activity, then the warm up becomes even more important.

A night of sleeping will increase the amount of fluid within the spinal discs. *This means if you are going to experience an issue with a disc, it is more likely to occur first thing in the morning.*

If you are working out later in the day, consider what you have been doing throughout the day. Are you at the office or in school? Has it been a day of sitting or inactivity? During this time, the body has likely been in a period of prolonged poor (slouched) posture. This is setting up the spine for injury. Sitting puts a very large load on the spine and in particular, the discs. Now combine this with hours of sitting. Your lumbar tissues are set up to fail. The warm up becomes even more critical the more inactive you have been (either due to sleep or sedentary behavior).

An adequate **warm up** should **always** be performed to help minimize the risk of injury and maximize your ability to perform the task or exercise.

Cardiovascular Warm Up

To properly prepare the body for activity, the first stage of the warm up is to increase blood flow throughout the body, but in particular, to the core muscles and spine. I recommend approximately 10 minutes as this allows for better mobility in the joints and tissues of the body. It starts to prime the nervous system for activity. It also promotes healing as movement is necessary to bring in the nutrients necessary to heal (if there is already damage or an injury).

The cardiovascular warm up will vary and is dependent on your activity or sport. When warming up for CrossFit or weightlifting, I like to use the stationary bike or the rower (as shown on the following page) for a 3-5 minutes before progressing to a more weight bearing activity, such as jogging, jump roping or any other form of standing movement (jumping, bounding, and jumping jacks), in order to increase my heart rate.

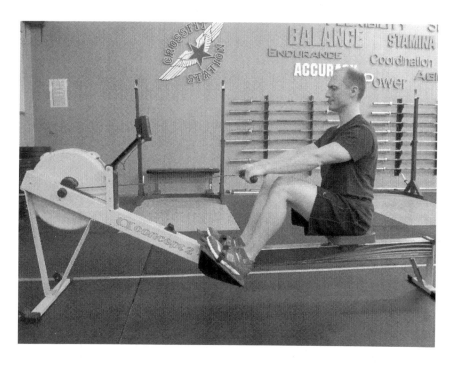

If I will be participating in a running event, then I will typically start by performing a light jog or possibility some jumping jacks. Then I may progress into some more intense heart rate increasing exercises, such as jump roping or any other form of standing movement (jumping, bounding, and burpees), in order to increase my heart rate. The goal is to increase your heart rate and promote blood flow body wide as you prime your body for exercise, so the warm up shouldn't be overly intense.

Dynamic Warm Up

After my initial cardiovascular warm up, I progress into my dynamic warm up series. This will typically involve warming up the muscles and joints of the spine, pelvis, and lower legs. (*This principle holds true for any upper body work. I would also perform a dynamic warm up of the shoulder girdle and upper thoracic area if I was preparing for exercise which involved my arms being overhead.)*

The purpose of the dynamic warm up (specifically in the lower extremity) is to insure adequate mobility in the areas that will be involved in the activity. This will almost always include the hamstrings, hips, and pelvis. Adequate lower leg mobility is important in order to perform your specific exercise or activity. The more motion that can occur through the pelvis and legs, the more force can then be generated and passed through the pelvis. More mobility in the lower legs and pelvis means less need for mobility in the spine. This means less stress during motion will be placed on the spine—therefore, decreasing your risk of injury. We want to maximize spinal stability and encourage movement through the hips, pelvis, and upper thoracic.

This also insures that adequate range of motion (ROM) can occur for your activity. *A risk factor for LBP is improper technique. If you don't have the available ROM to perform an activity or exercise, then you cannot perform it with the proper technique.*

During the warm up, I recommend that you **do not** perform any static stretching. It has been shown to decrease performance and may also increase the risk of injury. Any activity that is performed to improve mobility will either be via tissue mobilization (such as utilizing a foam roller) or with more dynamic activities. Stretching should only be performed post workout.

Within the dynamic warm up, you would perform exercises such as: forward and backward leg swings; side to side leg swings; squat with rotation; inchworm wiggle walkout push-up hop; forward bend and twist (to the easy side) to increase hamstrings length; split leg forward bend with rotation (to easy side); scorpion stretch; and press-ups.

If you are preparing for running or sports that involve running, you would perform exercises such as butt kickers, strides or bounding or sport specific drills (as well as any of the other listed exercises above).

Not every exercise mentioned needs to be performed each time. You may have some exercises you prefer over others, so find what works for you. Your goal is to have the whole system warm and mobile with an emphasis of the pelvis area (particularly, the glutes and hamstrings). *This would be the same for the shoulder girdle and upper thoracic area for overhead activities.* You may utilize the foam roller as part of a warm up, but as mentioned don't perform static stretching as it has been shown to decrease force production and performance.

Foam Roller

Utilizing a foam roller in addition to a dynamic warm up is an excellent method to address tightness in the lower leg, pelvis, and spine. It primes the tissues and nervous system for activity. Care should be taken. If there is an injury present, don't roll too aggressively. **How to use the foam roller:**

- I typically recommend one to three minutes of body weight rolling (if it is tolerated) per extremity, and the same for the thoracic, low back, and buttock area.

- A good rule of thumb is to roll out an area that is tender and sore or recently worked, until it no longer feels tight and sore.

- Again, approximately one to three minutes per area although this may vary based on your size. Increased time will be needed the more developed your muscles are.

- Initially begin by addressing any specific areas of tightness from the legs to the spine or those areas that tend to be a chronic issue for you.

- Foam rolling is generally not advised for those taking blood thinning medications or with blood clotting disorders.

- Avoid aggressive use of the foam roller in the case of acute and/or severe injury.

Lower Extremity Mobilizations using the Foam Roller

IT Band Mobilization with Foam Roller

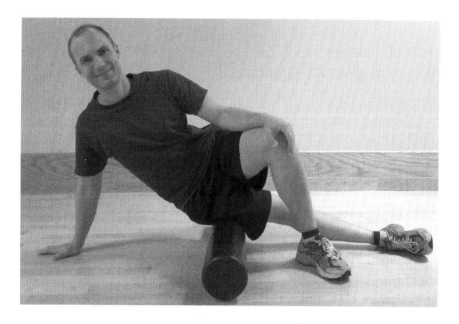

» Slowly roll your body back and forth along the entire length of the IT band and lateral thigh. Do not roll it over the greater trochanter of the hip (the boney part near your pelvis). Spend extra time on the most painful areas.

» Perform 1-2 minutes on each leg once per day.

Glutes and Buttock Mobilization

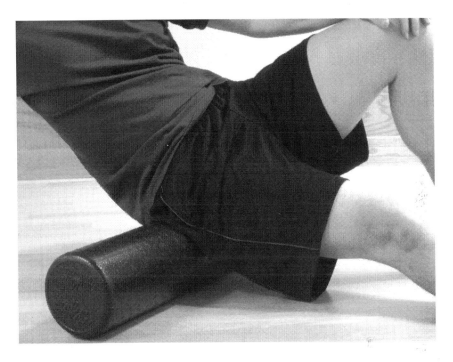

» Slowly roll your body back and forth along the buttock region. Continue on down the leg in the hamstring area as you feel it is needed. Spend extra time on the most painful areas.

» Perform 1-2 minutes on each leg once per day.

Hamstring Mobilization using the Foam Roller

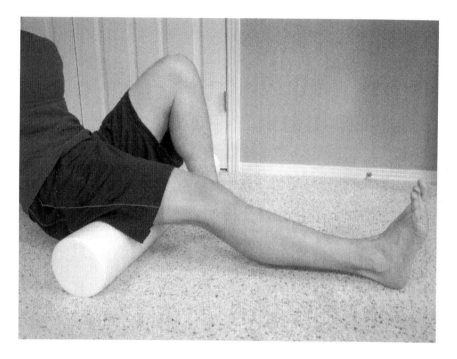

» Roll your hamstring back and forth on the foam roll. Move slowly and spend extra time on the more painful areas. Be sure to mobilize the entire hamstring and feel free to work on other areas of the leg that feel tight or restricted. If this is painful, do not exceed a mild to moderate amount of pain.

» Perform for 1-2 minutes per hamstring.

Quadriceps Mobilization

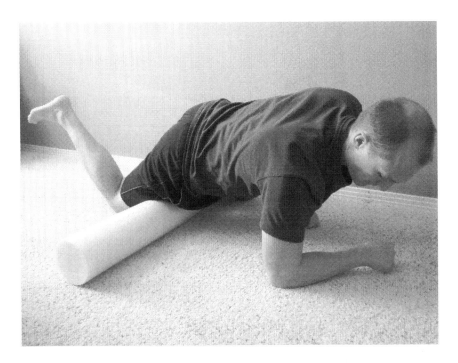

» Position your upper thigh onto the foam roller. You may have one or two legs on the roller. Slowly roll your body back and forth in order to cover the entire surface of the quadriceps. You may perform with both legs at a time or just one. Start with a straight leg. For added intensity, bend your knee. Spend extra time on the most painful areas.

» Perform 1-2 minutes on each leg once per day.

Quadriceps "Tack and Floss" Mobilization

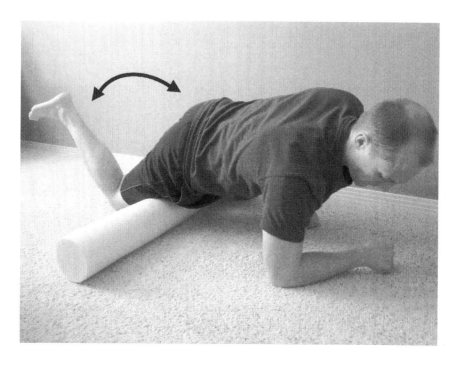

» Position your upper thigh onto the foam roller. Roll around until you locate a particularly tight and/or restricted area, and then very slowly bend your knee back and forth. Use the weight of your leg to hold the spasming muscle down over the foam roller as you slowly move back and forth over the foam roller by bending your knee.

» Perform 1-2 minutes on each leg once per day.

Spine Specific Warm Up

I am a big proponent to performing a very specific spinal muscle warm up upon completion of the cardiovascular and dynamic warm ups. Since you likely have already experienced an episode of LBP, a very specific and thorough warm up is important for prevention. Priming the specific muscles of the core (particularly, the multifidus and lumbar extensors) is a critical step to avoiding re-injury.

The multifidus is a critical muscle in preventing LBP and must be active to properly stabilize the spine. It helps to prevent shearing forces from affecting the spine. In the presence of pain, the multifidus muscle will actually shrink in size and doesn't fully return in size or strength without specific training. This is a reflexive action that occurs with injury or pain. (Similar muscle reflexes can be found in other muscle groups in the body. A common example is the quadriceps muscle, which will shrink and atrophy with knee injury or surgery.) Activating the multifidus muscle prior to exercise allows the muscle to activate and promotes increased blood flow in the area.

The theory is twofold. Like other muscle groups, you want to specifically activate them at a lower level as you increase the intensity of the exercise and activity. For example, you would never attempt a max squat without multiple warm up sets.

Secondly, spinal stability has many aspects to it. One specific portion is how the multifidus muscles work in combination with the transversus abdominis (TVA) muscle to help pull the thoracolumbar fascia and make an internal corset. You can increase the "tightness" of this internal corset by increasing the size of the lumbar extensor and specifically, the multifidus muscles. This is performed via the "muscle pump." Muscles get bigger after exercise as they are engorged with blood. Use this to your advantage with the multifidus by performing a few sets of exercise to insure they are ready to work. This also increases blood flow to the area which helps to increase your body's ability to make an internal corset for spinal stability. It also primes the nervous system to insure proper muscle firing (both timing and force of contraction). However, don't work the muscles to the point of fatigue. You want them fresh and ready to work throughout your activity and exercise.

Regardless of your training or event time and/or location, don't skip the warm up. You may be the only one performing a thorough warm up, but you understand the importance of the warm up in order to prevent LBP and to improve your performance.

I recently participated in a Spartan obstacle race. We were in the middle of nowhere, but I still went through my warm up routine which included getting face down in the dirt and weeds to perform my press-ups and multifidus activation series. Later that day, I heard that multiple participants hurt their backs during the stone medicine ball carry. Lesson learned. I didn't see hardly anyone warming up prior to the event. Perform your warm up. It really does matter!

Specific Lumbar Warm Up Exercises

My recommended exercises to activate the multifidus muscles include the following superman exercises and bridging. I typically advise 10-20 repetitions each. Use these in conjunction with press-ups, which help to improve mobility and prepare the area for activity.

Superman Exercise – Starting Position

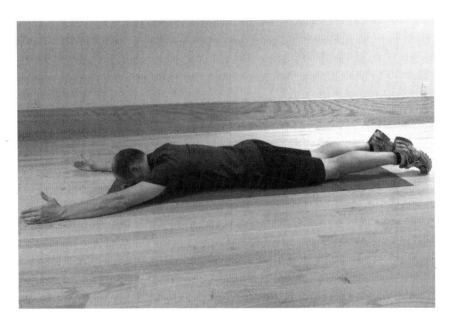

» Lie on the ground with your arms stretched out in a "V" position. Support your head with a small rolled up towel to maintain a neutral spine, and keep your chin slightly tucked.

» You can lie on the floor or a bed. If you are on a bed, you may need a pillow under your stomach for extra support and comfort.

Superman Exercise – Legs

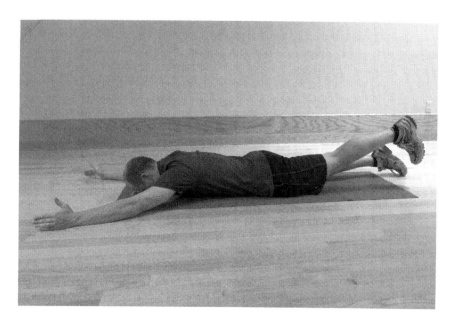

» Raise one leg at a time while being sure to keep your abdominal muscles active. Don't arch your back. Raise your leg up 4-6 inches if you can. If you start to twist in the trunk or low back, then stop. Only raise the leg as far as you can without twisting.

» Perform 1 set of 10 repetitions prior to activity.

Superman Exercise – Arms and Legs (Opposite)

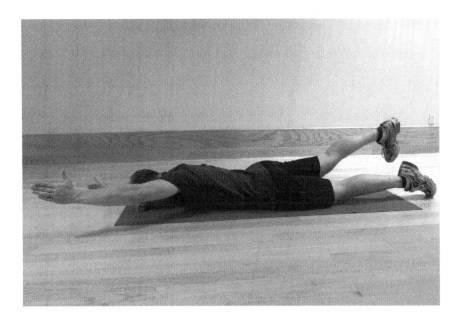

» Raise your opposite arm and leg. Be sure to keep your abdominal muscles active. Don't arch your back. Raise your leg up 4-6 inches if you can. If you start to twist in the trunk or low back, then stop. Only raise the leg as far as you can without twisting. Be sure to keep your chin slightly tucked and in a neutral position. Keep your shoulder blades back and down. Don't shrug.

» Perform 1 set of 10 repetitions prior to activity.

Superman Exercise – Arms and Legs (Same Time)

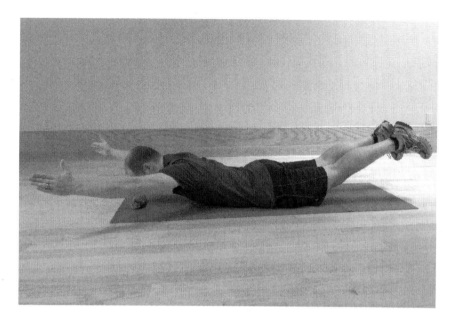

» Raise your arms and legs. Be sure to keep your abdominal muscles active. Don't over arch your back. Raise your legs up 4-6 inches if you can. As your head elevates, be sure to keep your chin slightly tucked and in a neutral position. Keep your shoulder blades back and down.

» Perform 2 sets of 10 repetitions prior to activity.

Bridge Exercise – Starting Position

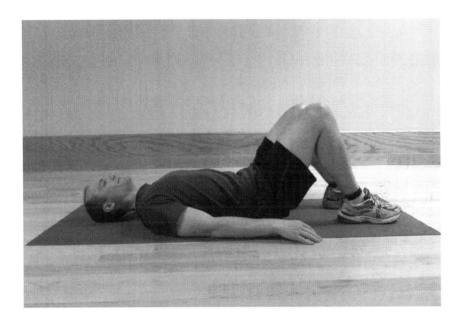

» Lie on your back with your knees bent to prepare for the bridge exercise.

Bridge Exercise

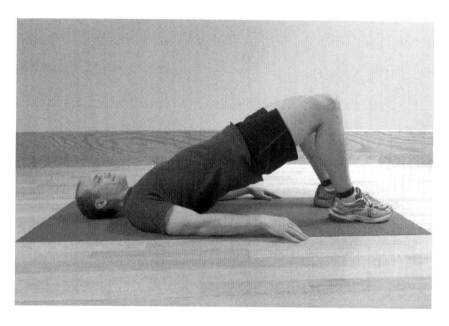

» Keep your pelvis level as you lift your hips/pelvis and buttocks into the air. Pause, and then return back down to the ground. Do not let your pelvis wobble as you move up and down. Add a weight to your pelvis to increase the difficulty level.

» Perform 2 sets of 10 repetitions prior to activity.

Bridge Exercise with Straight Leg Raise

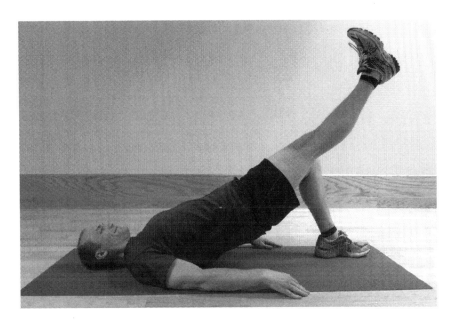

» Keep your pelvis level as you lift your hips/pelvis and buttocks into the air. Pause, extend your leg. Hold for 3-5 seconds, then return the leg to the ground and repeat with the opposite leg. Return your buttocks to the ground and rest when you can no longer keep your pelvis from wobbling or your buttocks from dropping downward. Perform on both legs.

» Perform 2 sets of 10 repetitions prior to activity.

Activity Specific Warm Up

This is when you actually perform the activity or exercise that you will be participating in, but with a lighter load or decreased intensity. If the activity is weightlifting, use just enough weight to allow you to properly perform the movement, such as using an empty bar, when performing a power clean or use an empty bar while performing several squats.

The goal is to insure that your body is ready to perform the desired activity through a complete and total range of motion (ROM) without tightness and restriction. If you feel tight, restricted or in any way not ready, then return to the initial warm up (cardiovascular or dynamic). Your body should feel absolutely ready prior to starting the activity.

If you are ready to proceed, initially begin slowly and then progress to full speed or intensity. This principle holds true for all activities including sprinting. In this case, get down in the starting blocks. Practice your initial take off and sprint 10-20 yards before returning to the blocks and repeating. Depending on the sport, break down a few select movement patterns. Perform just those patterns at full speed. An example may be a full speed fast break layup for basketball or side to side cutting drills for soccer or football. Tailor your warm up to your specific event. The cardiovascular and dynamic warm up will be similar for everyone, but the activity specific warm up will be different as it is sport specific.

Weightlifters: If you are performing activities that require a lot of bending, then you may choose to utilize standing back extensions before and after your work sets. This becomes even more important if you have a history of LBP due to flexion related activity or if you typically spend a most of your day either bending over or sitting. Don't sit for any length of time in between sets. Be up standing or preferably, walking. Don't worry, your legs will recover between sets whether you sit or stand and walk.

This warm up sequence can seem a bit tedious since it includes: a cardiovascular warm up; a dynamic warm up; a spine specific warm up; and an activity or sport specific warm up. However, when performed properly, this should only take approximately 15-20 minutes. The benefits of a regular and thorough warm up are huge. You will reduce your risk of injury (spinal or otherwise). You will also find that you can significantly increase the intensity and effectiveness of your workouts which allows for greater training success. *Nothing derails a perfectly programmed training routine faster than an injury.*

THE COOL DOWN

After performing your activity, take the extra time to cool down and stretch. A stationary bike at a causal/slower pace or rower are great options. Both are reduced weight bearing exercises that promote movement and circulation to the knee as well as work on lower extremity ROM. Walking is also always a good option. You want to keep moving at least long enough for your heart rate to return close to baseline.

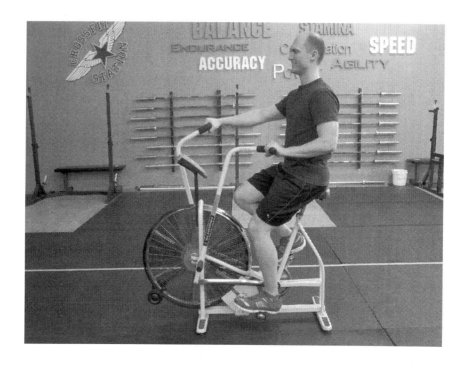

Self-Mobilize

Utilizing the foam roller or other self-mobilization tools also works well as part of your cool down. This should not be performed until your heart rate has recovered.

Reasons to utilize the foam roller include:

- Highly recommended for athletic performance.

- It appears it can help improve joint ROM.

- It does not impede performance.

- It can likely help with recovery either by reducing soreness or reducing post work out tightness. It promotes improved blood flow which allows for improved nutrient delivery that can improve recovery times.

- Improving recovery may allow for more intense or frequent training sessions or prepare you for multiple events with little rest.

- Sometimes eliminating soreness prior to activity can have a psychological boost which shouldn't be overlooked as an important outcome.

How to use the foam roller:

- I typically recommend one to three minutes of body weight rolling (if it is tolerated) per extremity, and the same for the thoracic, low back, and buttock area.

- A good rule of thumb is to roll out an area that is tender and sore or recently worked, until it no longer feels tight and sore.

- Again, approximately one to three minutes per area although this may vary based on your size. Increased time will be needed the more developed your muscles are.

- Foam rolling is generally not advised for those taking blood thinning medications or with blood clotting disorders.

For specific instructions, please refer to **Lower Extremity Mobilizations using the Foam Roller.**

Static Stretching

Static stretching should be implemented as part of your cool down. This is the perfect time to stretch the muscles that were used most during the activity just performed. It is also the perfect time to work on those tight and chronically restricted areas. The tissues tend to respond best to stretching at the end of session when the body is still warm, but when any risk of decreasing performance has passed. Immediately sitting down after intense exercise or weightlifting increases your risk of developing back pain. Take the cool down seriously. Please refer to **Leg and Pelvic Stretches for Low Back Pain**.

LOW BACK PAIN (LBP)
PREVENTION STRATEGIES

CROSS TRAINING

Performing the same activity day after day without variation can lead to overuse injuries or muscle imbalances. You will spend a majority of your time training on your particular sport or activity. It's important to vary the training load and/or stimulus. This can limit your risk of injury. Not only can cross training be fun, but it keeps the body stimulated and ready to improve. The goal of cross training for LBP prevention is to insure varied stimulus and load throughout the body. This will help the body develop more completely to be more symmetrically strong and stable. Often, weakness in a leg or a hip muscle will cause a person to compensate in some way. This compensation can change normal mechanics and alignment of the spine and lower body while increasing the risk of injury.

SPOT TRAINING

To limit your risk of injury, address any areas of weakness that may lead to inappropriate movements or compensation patterns. This will also limit your risk of injuring other parts of the body that may be involved in the compensation patterns. Like in cross training, the goal is to help the body develop more fully and symmetrically. First, identify the weak areas, the areas that are chronically tight, and the areas where mobility is restricted. Then work on those specific areas.

For instance, a weak core and weak pelvic muscles are a common issue among runners. This weakness causes abnormal loading patterns in the lower leg. Hip and core weakness is one of the major risk factors for knee pain.

Also, if you have weak hamstrings, lifting a load from the ground will cause you to rely on more lumbar and glutes activation. The hamstrings are not contributing enough force. This increases the risk of injury to the hamstrings and also to the low back.

Do your knees roll in during a heavy squat or a one leg jump? If so, likely your hip muscles are weak. As part of your cool down, implement exercises to help work on those areas that need specific attention. You may need to focus some training time on the area in addition to your cool down. Please refer to **Core Strengthening Exercises – Lumbar Extensors**.

ACHES AND PAIN

Be proactive. Don't wait to manage those aches and pains! Most of the time you will be able to self-treat. Get regular body work from a masseuse. Use your foam roller. Spot train your weak areas, and work on whole body mobility and fitness. Don't neglect the small stuff. It will catch up with you sooner or later. Address potential issues early for a quicker resolution and to prevent little things from becoming major injuries that derail your training for weeks or months.

Many aches and pains are actually caused by faulty mechanics from weak areas or mobility related issues elsewhere. Although treating the actual areas that are sore and tender is important, you will need to identify the cause of the soreness. These sore areas or "hot spots" are sending a warning signal that your body is not functioning as well as it should. Be proactive in identifying the areas that need additional support and work, and continue with your spot training. Sometimes you may have to ask for help in identifying the true culprits. It's always easier to address these areas early rather than wait for a catastrophic injury that would completely derail your training plans.

MODIFY THE ACTIVITY

If it hurts, don't do it! If the activity is causing you pain, then you will need to modify the activity or discontinue it completely. It's okay to modify any exercise as needed. Don't compromise proper technique to complete an exercise. This also holds true for range of motion (ROM). If you don't have adequate ROM to perform the activity with a low load, then definitely don't attempt it under a high load or under a higher velocity. That will significantly increase your risk of injury. Work with your coach. Often, poor form and technique is the cause of the pain. With additional instruction, you can avoid pain and injury and take your training to the next level.

ADEQUATE REST

Your body must rest in order to grow and develop. Training seven days a week is not the best way to improve. Instead, it can lead to injury and burn out. Take a rest day. Do something fun. It can still be active such as a yoga class, a leisurely bike ride or a walk in the park. If you are working with a yearly training cycle, be sure to implement an off season that involves a change of pace from your regular training and some active rest. Proper programming includes mini cycles with an off season as well as active rest cycles in between heavy load and heavy volume training cycles. Your rest and recovery days should be as intentional as your training days.

RECOVERY PROTOCOL

Be specific and strategic about your recovery protocol. Overtraining increases your risk of injury. A recovery protocol should include a multifaceted approach that implements strategies to positively affect the muscular, nervous, and hormonal systems. Many of these strategies are performed post exercise as part of a programmed recovery. Don't skip this vital component to injury prevention! You will also find that an adequate recovery will allow for a more intense training session the next time. In almost all cases, quality will trump quantity. Adequate recovery allows for each training session to be high quality.

HOW TO SELF-TREAT LOW BACK PAIN (LBP) FOLLOWING AN INJURY

INITIAL TREATMENT

Sometimes it is obvious when an injury to the lumbar spine has occurred. Other times the pain is much more subtle. The pain can start slowly increasing throughout the day until you are in a full blown case of low back pain.

To safely self-treat your low back pain, first take a moment to assess your symptoms and pain level. What led to your pain and/or injury? Did the pain come on suddenly or slowly? Evaluate the severity of the injury. **If you're experiencing any of the following, please seek immediate medical attention:**

- Loss of bowel/bladder function.

- Uncontrollable pain. The pain is so severe you cannot function or move.

- Ataxia (a neurological sign) occurs when you are unable to control or coordinate the movements in your legs (particularly, during walking).

- You are losing muscle function or control. The muscles in the legs will no longer work. (This is different than pain preventing the muscle from working.) This sensation of paralysis occurs when the muscles will not actually function.

- Significant loss of sensation in the leg or groin area. This is not a tingling sensation, but an actual loss of sensation. For example, you cannot feel the toilet paper when you wipe after using the toilet.

- Numbness, pins and needles or severe pain in the toes or lower leg.

- The pain does not change with movement or worsens with rest.

- Any history of cancer or tumor, and the pain did not have a specific and correlated mechanism for injury.

- Onset of pain without any known mechanism for the injury. (Thoroughly consider your activity. Many times, a slow onset of pain begins several hours after performing an activity.)

- If you also develop a high fever or any other symptoms in relation to your low back pain or generally start not feeling well.

DIRECTIONAL PREFERENCE

- Because most LBP is mechanical, you should be able to alter and change it within a short period of time. Most LBP will have a directional preference for extension, meaning extending backward. A majority of injuries occur either performing a forward biased (flexed movement) or are due to chronic slouching (a forward biased or spinal flexion biased movement).

- First, establish a directional preference. This means establish a pattern to the pain. Does it get worse when you bend over or better? What happens when you repeat this movement?

- Determine how the pain responds. If it spreads away from the spine and down into the leg, beware that you are moving in the wrong direction. Stop that particular movement, and instead try moving in the opposite direction. If you were moving into flexion, try extension. If you had trialed extension biased movements, try flexion.

Fortunately, most LBP is mechanical--meaning it is from a physical or structural cause and isn't related to conditions such as cancer or infections. Most LBP will have a directional preference for extension. A majority of injuries occur when performing a forward biased (flexed movement) like chronic slouching or a spinal flexion biased movement. Flexion biased programs are often found in older adults (particularly in cases of spinal stenosis). They may also be seen in younger clients suffering from a specific type of spinal fracture known as a spondylolisthesis. Please refer to **Special Topics**.

You should be able to alter and change your LBP within a short period of time. First, establish a directional preference by identifying a pattern to the pain. Does the pain get worse when you bend over or does it improve? What happens when you repeat this movement? Determine how your pain responds. If it spreads away from the spine and down into the leg, beware that you are moving in the wrong direction. Stop that particular movement, and instead try flexion biased movements. In my experience, most episodes of LBP tend to respond better to extension biased movements. If flexion or extension doesn't help or change the pain in any way, then you may need assistance from a medical provider.

The rule of thumb for movement:

If the pain worsens by spreading peripherally down the buttock and into the leg and/or foot, then the condition is worsening. We must stop that activity. If the pain centralizes and returns back toward the spine (even if the pain worsens slightly), then keep moving as the condition is actually improving. For a thorough discussion and an excellent treatment resource, please refer to *Treat Your Own Back* by Robin A. McKenzie.

SELF-TREATMENT STRATEGIES

Although most LBP isn't considered serious, the pain tends to re-occur. One major reason for this is that the deep stabilizing muscles, known as the **multifidus muscles**, reflexively shrink, weaken, and lose function. Without proper rehabilitation, the muscles will not fully recover. This increases the risk of future episodes because the spine no longer has the ability to stabilize itself normally. Initially after a suspected injury, I highly advise that you don't sit. Instead, keep moving, but slowly.

If you have established your directional preference as an **extension biased**, I typically recommend performing press-ups and standing back extensions. Please refer to **Extension Biased Stretches for Low Back Pain**.

If you have established your directional preference as **flexion biased**, I typically recommend performing the following exercises: knee to chest, double knee to chest, and seated flexion. Please refer to **Flexion Biased Stretches for Low Back Pain.**

- **ACTIVATE THE MULTIFIDUS.** *Other than determining directional preference, and then performing the associated exercises this is the <u>most important</u> component to treatment.* Start with spine extensor muscle activation (the muscles that extend your spine) exercises such as the superman and bridging (as demonstrated in **Core Strengthening Exercises – Lumbar Extensors**). Perform these exercises frequently during the day after the initial injury. Once the pain subsides and muscle function improves, more advanced lumbar extension strengthening and stabilizing exercises will need to be performed to decrease your risk of recurrent low back pain.

  These exercises are listed from easiest to hardest. Begin with the prone (on your stomach) superman exercises and bridging exercises. **At all times, follow the rule of peripheralization and centralization.** If your pain progresses from the area of the injury into your leg, then you need to stop that activity. If the pain remains constant or is progressing out of the leg, then continue with the activity as you are helping the body to heal. The key to long term management is a strong core (particularly, the multifidus and posterior chain muscles).

- **DON'T SIT.** Walking is critical to your recovery! It's the number one way your spine receives nutrients and disposes of metabolic waste products. Walk frequently, and try to avoid any prolonged sitting. This is a critical component to spine health. Walk more!

- **IF YOU SIT, USE PROPER POSTURE.** Utilize a **McKenzie lumbar roll** to help insure a correct lumbar curve *(as shown on page 31)*. Be sure to get up every 20-30 minutes. If you cannot comfortably sit, then listen to your body.

- **REDUCE INFLAMMATION AND SUPPORT THE HEALING RESPONSE.** I recommend starting a 30 day course of **CapraFlex by Mt. Capra.** CapraFlex is an organic glucosamine and chondroitin supplement which also includes an herbal and spice formulation designed to naturally decrease inflammation and support healing. I recommend it to anyone recovering from an injury or attempting to prevent injury when performing at a very high level. I personally use it, and in my practice, it has helped clients recover faster and prevent injury.

  Tissue Rejuvenator by Hammer Nutrition contains glucosamine and chondroitin as well as a host of herbs, spices, and enzymes to help support tissues and limit inflammation. I recommend taking either CapraFlex **OR** Tissue Rejuvenator. I typically recommend trying a 14-30 day protocol.

  An additional supplement to consider is called **CapraColostrum by Mt. Capra.** Colostrum is the first milk produced by female mammals after giving birth. It contains a host of immunoglobulins, anti-microbial peptides, and other growth factors. It is especially good at strengthening the intestinal lining which prevents and heals conditions associated with a leaky gut. Colostrum can also help a person more effectively exercise in hotter conditions. Over all, it can boost the immune system, assist with intestinal issues, and help the body to recover faster.

I recommend taking either CapraFlex **OR** Tissue Rejuvenator, not both concurrently. You **can** take CapraColostrum independently or in conjunction with either CapraFlex or Tissue Rejuvenator.

If the supplements are aiding in your recovery, you may choose to continue taking them for an additional 30 days. I sometimes implement this protocol as part of a prevention strategy during times of heavy volume or high intensity training.

Please consult with your pharmacist and/or physician prior to starting any new supplementation protocol. Herbs could interact with some medications particularly if you are taking blood thinners.

- **ICE AS NEEDED FOR PAIN.** *The rule for icing is to apply ice no more than twenty minutes per hour.* Do not place the ice directly against the skin, especially if you are using a gel pack style. *Individuals with poor circulation or impaired sensation should take particular care when icing.* The ice is for pain control only. It doesn't penetrate deep enough into your back to affect any of the likely pain generating structures.

After the first few days, you can alternate between applying heat or ice (depends on your amount of relief from either). The protocol for only using ice for the first two weeks is not so strict when treating LBP. Typically, the rule on more superficial injuries, such as a shoulder injury or ankle sprain, is to ice for two weeks.

Individuals with poor circulation or impaired sensation should take particular care when icing.

- **USE TOPICAL ANALGESICS FOR PAIN.** There are many topical agents which can be used for pain. My two favorites to help manage pain and stiffness are **Arnica Rub** (an herbal rub) and **Biofreeze**. Use liberally. These help with pain, but they don't get to the source of the pain. In addition to icing, use these topicals as tools to get moving more in order to help the injury heal faster.

- **BE AS ACTIVE AS YOU CAN.** Don't stop moving! It's important that you remain as active as you can, but taper back on certain activities that you know will increase your pain. This typically would be activities that involve heavy loading of the spine or excessive use of the piriformis muscle such as squats with weight, deadlifts or other activities that may cause forward flexion (particularly under a load or standing on one leg).

As you are able, continue to work on cardiovascular conditioning and core muscle activation, particularly the lumbar extensors. Remember the rule of thumb for movement. If your pain progresses from the area of injury into the leg, then you need to stop that activity. If the pain remains constant or is progressing out of the leg, then continue with the activity as you are helping the body to heal.

- **HYDRATE.** The human body is primarily made of water, which is critical for all body functions. I highly encourage you to hydrate more frequently during recovery. Adequate water intake is critical as your body attempts to heal and flush out metabolic wastes. Dehydrated tissues are prone to injury as they struggle to gain needed nutrients to heal and repair. Dehydrated tissues are less flexible and tend to accumulate waste products. Maintain a steady supply of nutrients going to/from the area of the injury. Try to avoid beverages that contain artificial sweeteners or chemicals with names you can't spell or pronounce. Water is best.

- **ORAL MAGNESIUM. Although** you can increase the magnesium in your diet by eating foods higher in magnesium such as spinach, artichokes, and dates, I recommend that you take **Mag Glycinate** in pill form. Taking additional magnesium (particularly at night) can help to reduce muscle cramps and spasming. It is also very helpful in reducing overall muscle soreness and aiding in a better night's rest. I recommend beginning with a dose of 200 mg (before bedtime) and increasing the dose as needed. I would caution you that taking too much magnesium can lead to diarrhea. Mag Glycinate in its oral form is the most highly absorbable. Although not as absorbable, **Thorne Research Magnesium Citrate** and magnesium oxide can also be beneficial.

- **ACUPUNCTURE.** I am personally a big fan of acupuncture. It's very useful in treating all kinds of medical conditions. It can be particularly effective in treating muscle cramps and spasms as it addresses the issues on multiple layers. Acupuncture directly stimulates the muscle by affecting the nervous system response to the muscle while producing a general sense of well-being and relaxation.

- **BRACING.** A lumbar corset brace may also be worn initially after injury. This works just like the thoracolumbar fascia—it helps to support and stabilize the spine. It also acts as a reminder to avoid flexing. You will want to wear it snug. This should only be a temporary measure. Frequent use of the brace will further weaken your body's own lumbar stabilizing muscles. The brace is only worn initially for pain relief. As soon as possible, discontinue the brace. Continue working through the proper extension or flexion biased movements while working on core strengthening.

- **ASK FOR HELP.** Yes, even physical therapists have to ask for help sometimes! Many useful manual and manipulation based techniques can help to manage LBP, particularly when combined with the right exercise and movement based protocol. Most manual techniques cannot be performed on your own.

If your pain isn't improving, seek a qualified and competent physical therapist or sports chiropractor who specializes in working with athletic clients who suffer from low back pain. One test to see if the practitioner is a good fit is to ask his/her advice on using manual techniques and exercise. If the practitioner doesn't believe in movement and exercise based treatment in combination with manual therapy, keep looking. **The American Physical Therapy Association** offers a wonderful resource to help find a physical therapist in your area. In most states, you can seek physical therapy advice without a medical doctor's referral (although it may be a good idea to seek your physician's opinion as well).

LOW BACK PAIN (LBP) POST ACUTE TREATMENT

This portion of your recovery is usually several days to over a week post injury. You have already been working through the initial treatment including: establishing a directional preference; limiting sitting; staying active; and starting a basic core activation program. Now that the pain has somewhat subsided, it's time to get into the specifics of your rehabilitation. It's primarily directed at core and lumbar extensor strengthening and addressing any issues that may predispose you to injury. Throughout this process, you will likely continue on many of the treatments utilized during the initial treatment such as applying icing and topical agents while limiting sitting and avoiding poor posture.

The following exercises and rehabilitation strategies are demon-strated in the **Low Back Pain (LBP) – Rehabilitation Guide**.

- **ACTIVATE THE MULTIFIDUS.** This is a critical component to your treatment and prevention strategy. Once the pain subsides and muscle function improves, more advanced lumbar extension strengthening and stabilizing exercises should be performed to decrease your risk of re-current LBP. Do not progress to more advanced exercises until the initial activation exercises (such as the superman and standard bridge) can be performed easily and relatively pain free.

Continue to progress through these exercises by adding repetitions and increasing the difficulty level. As pain subsides and function improves, progress into exercises such as straight leg dead lifts and dead lifts. You can also add weight when performing back extensions over the exercise ball. There are many different exercise combinations. Until you can properly perform the good morning exercise, don't progress into the straight leg dead lifts. For more ideas, please refer to **Core Strengthening and Full Body Exercises – Emphasis on Lumbar Extensors**.

If available in your area, utilize a lumbar extension machine known as the **Lumbar MedX**. It's probably the single best lumbar extensor exercise.

- **STRETCH THE MUSCLES OF THE LEGS AND PELVIS.** Stretching the hamstrings, hip flexors, and piriformis muscles daily helps to reduce muscle spasms and tightness throughout pelvis area. Poor pelvic and hip mobility causes excessive strain in the lumbar spine and can lead to improper movement patterns particularly when exercising. If you spend any portion of your day sitting, implementing a stretching and mobility protocol as a prevention strategy and recovery is critical. I typically stretch for at least 30 seconds at a time, and two to three times each session (and even longer for the hamstrings). Please refer to **Leg and Pelvic Stretches for Low Back Pain**.

- **INITIATE A HIP/PELVIC STRENGTHENING PRO-GRAM.** Once the initial severe pain has subsided and you have been practicing the lumbar strengthening program, it's time to add exercises that specifically target the piriformis muscle, gluteus medius, and other hip rotators and stabilizers. If you choose your exercises correctly, you can also implement more lumbar extensor strengthening into your routine at the same time. Consider exercises such as **single leg bridging** and **bridging with an exercise band** around your knees.

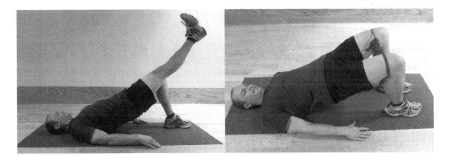

You can also perform exercises such as **side stepping with an exercise band** around your knee.

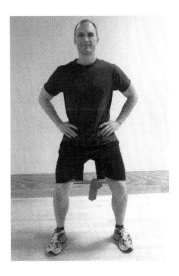

- **KINESIOLOGICAL TAPING.** Like the lumbar corset brace, Kinesiological taping techniques can be utilized to help support the lumbar spine. The taping can remind your body what directions not to move in and possibly facilitate muscle function. The tape can be worn as part of an initial treatment strategy, and the "H" technique can also be worn as a prevention strategy. To learn how to apply the Kinesiological tape, I have demonstrated both the star and "H" techniques in **Low Back Pain – Kinesiological Taping**. Please refer to **Skin Care with Taping** as well.

- **MASSAGE.** Contact a masseuse, physical therapist, athletic trainer or a friend who is skillful in body work and massage to relieve the painful area. The specific massage technique to use will vary according to your preference. Massage techniques range from a light relaxing massage to a deep tissue massage or utilization of acupressure points.

- **MOBILIZE THE TISSUE.** I highly recommend that you use the foam roller initially. For specific instructions, please refer to **Lower Extremity Mobilizations using the Foam Roller**. General guidelines include:

  - I typically recommend one to three minutes of body weight rolling (if it is tolerated) per extremity, and the same for the thoracic, low back, and buttock area.

  - A good rule of thumb is to roll out an area that is tender and sore or recently worked, until it no longer feels tight and sore.

- Again, approximately one to three minutes per area although this may vary based on your size. Increased time will be needed the more developed your muscles are.

- Foam rolling is generally not advised for those taking blood thinning medications or with blood clotting disorders.

As you can tolerate, progress to utilizing a **lacrosse ball to aggressively mobilize the piriformis muscle**. I tend to focus on smaller areas for a longer period of time. I recommend only a few minutes per area as you can easily overdo and cause more pain. The foam roller works best for larger areas while the lacrosse ball can pinpoint smaller harder to reach regions (particularly, in the buttocks).

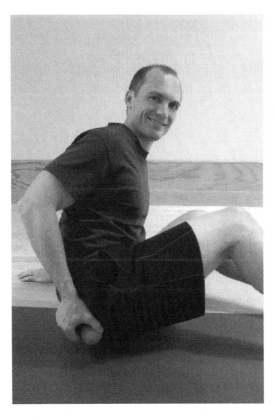

- **SUPPLEMENTATION.** Continue with your supplementation protocol (as addressed in **Self-Treatment Strategies**). This includes oral or topical magnesium supplementation as well as supplements to limit inflammation and support the healing response. I recommend taking a combination of **CapraFlex by Mt. Capra** OR **Tissue Rejuvenator by Hammer Nutrition** with **CapraColostrum by Mt. Capra**.

- **ASK FOR HELP.** Yes, even physical therapists have to ask for help sometimes! Many useful manual and manipulation based techniques can help to manage LBP, particularly when combined with the right exercise and movement based protocol. Most manual techniques cannot be performed on your own.

If your pain isn't improving, seek a qualified and competent physical therapist or sports chiropractor who specializes in working with athletic clients who suffer from low back pain. One test to see if the practitioner is a good fit is to ask his/her advice on using manual techniques and exercise. If the practitioner doesn't believe in movement and exercise based treatment in combination with manual therapy, keep looking. **The American Physical Therapy Association** offers a wonderful resource to help find a physical therapist in your area. In most states, you can seek physical therapy advice without a medical doctor's referral (although it may be a good idea to seek your physician's opinion as well).

SPECIAL TOPICS

In this particular section, I address special topics and conditions in relation to low back pain (LBP) and injury. Although there are many more spinal related conditions and injuries, the following are the most common conditions that many of my clients suffer from.

SPONDYLOLISTHESIS (SPONDY)

Spondylolisthesis (also referred to as spondy, or a pars defect) is a certain kind of back injury that is associated with a pars interarticularis defect which is part of the vertebrae. This condition can be congenital (from birth) or happen from trauma. It is diagnosed slightly more in males (5% of the male population versus 3% in the female population).

It is important to note if the fracture is stable or not. If the spondylolisthesis is unstable during active motion, such as bending forward or backward, the vertebrae can actually slip and move forward or backward.

Spondylolisthesis injuries are graded I, II, III, IV, and V.

- A Grade I defect occurs when 25% of the vertebral body has slipped forward.

- Grade II occurs when 50% of the vertebral body slips forward.

- Grade III occurs when 75% of the vertebral body slips forward.

- Grade IV occurs when 100% of the vertebral body slips forward.

- Grade V occurs when the vertebral body completely falls off which causes a spondyloptosis.

In many cases, you will never know if you have this particular condition unless an X-ray is taken. Many times, spondy is an incidental diagnosis. Meaning an x-ray or other imaging was performed due to complaints of low back pain, and then it was noticed on the imaging. Often, the pain is not correlated to the actual spondy diagnosis. Most of my recommended treatment plan and strategies are still helpful when dealing with spondylolisthesis.

If you have a Grade I or II spondylolisthesis, conservative treatment (including formal physical therapy) is usually the first form of treatment. Surgical intervention may be performed as needed in the case of a Grade II spondylolisthesis. Surgical or other medical intervention is almost always necessary in cases of Grade III or higher.

Exercise and Treatment Considerations

In case of a stable Grade I and some Grade II spondylolisthesis, exercise is an important part of the treatment strategy. There are a few items of consideration. First, obtain clearance from your medical physician. Often, a series of X-rays will be taken while you are standing and bending either forward or backward. This can determine if the area is stable.

Once you know that the area is stable, then you can treat the spine very similarly to my recommended treatment plan and strategies. Always let pain and directional preference guide your movements.

On average, I tend to have my clients be less aggressive with lumbar range of motion, especially press-ups and backward bending. Although it's not prohibited completely in the case of a stable injury, it's merely a precaution as some research indicates that it may have the potential to cause more pain and worsen the pars defect.

It is also entirely possible that the cause of pain has nothing to do with the spondylolisthesis. A thorough physical therapy evaluation should help to determine the actual cause of the pain (although, sometimes it is never truly known).

The focus of the treatment and exercise is on the strengthening of the inner and outer core muscles and lumbar extensors. With the only caveat being that you may need to avoid excessive loading with the spine extended. In this instance, I recommend that you work with a highly qualified trainer or sports medicine professional to insure that you are performing your particular exercise and sport in a manner that will keep you safe and the fracture stable.

It is also important to insure proper hip and pelvic mobility to insure that the spine is not over worked. In cases of spondylolis-thesis, insuring a normal amount of hip extension in addition to proper hamstring length and hip rotation is important. If the hip cannot fully extend during walking and running, it will cause excessive lumbar extension. You may even want to focus on having less of a lumbar curve (a posterior pelvic tilt) if your tendency is to hyper extend with an anterior pelvic tilt. Be sure to work on thoracic mobility to insure the entire vertebral chain can move freely.

Exercise is a critical component to the management of this condition. I would highly advise that you consult with a local physical therapist that has a **Lumbar MedX** exercise machine. This particular machine can isolate the lumbar multifidus during exercise better than any other exercise that I am aware of.

The **Core Strengthening Exercises – Lumbar Extensors** are designed to progressively activate the multifidus muscles (with the final exercise being the most challenging). When implementing these exercises, be sure to not over extend the spine and as with all conditions, monitor your symptoms. If you perform an activity that causes worsening pain, then you will need to modify or eliminate that particular activity until it can be performed pain free.

In some cases, more flexion biased stretches would be indicated. This would be determined by the directional preference. If extension biased exercises worsened the pain and flexion biased exercises improved the pain, then initially you would proceed with flexion biased exercises to help control pain while you progress into your core and lumbar stabilization program. Please refer to **Flexion Biased Stretches for Low Back Pain,** which includes the following exercises: knee to chest, double knee to chest, and seated flexion.

INSTABILITIES

Although most people (medical and otherwise) don't fully understand the concept, instability in the vertebrae of the spine is actually very common. Instabilities are usually diagnosed by a physical therapist or a chiropractor. Often, it will be described as a subluxation (or that something is out of place). Except for the case of a severe fracture, the spine doesn't dislocate (as could a shoulder).

Due to injury and poor muscle motor control, the movement of certain segments (vertebrae) within the spine can be more than others. At times, this can cause a mal-alignment. I like to use the analogy of a cross threaded lid. The lid needs to be line up properly to work when it is cross threaded. It's still a lid, but it may either be stuck on too tight or not be on tight enough. Either way, this will cause dysfunction and pain.

Like most spine related conditions, the best way to treat and manage spinal instabilies and the associated pain is through lumbar stabilization exercises. Please refer to the **Core Strengthening Exercises – Lumbar Extensors**.

Inner and outer core strength as well as a strong posterior chain will be a vital component to managing this type of condition. In addition to generally becoming stronger, insuring proper motor control during exercise is also important. The key is to focus on engaging the inner core prior to performing the exercise and activity.

DISC INJURIES

Although there are many different types of vertebral disc injuries, most will not require surgery. Healing can be a slow process, but many of these types of injuries will resolve. Some schools of thought feel that disc injuries of one form or another make up a large percentage of reports of low back pain (LBP). I am unsure if that is true based upon my research, but I will agree that in most cases, conservative treatment is the best option. There is definitely a time and place for surgical intervention.

My recommended self-treatment strategies can help those attempting to recover from a disc injury. Watching for the "red flag" symptoms (as noted in **Initial Treatment**) and following the directional preference rule works especially well when treating disc related injuries. Continue with my recommended exercise based approach. As symptoms resolve, focus on developing proper lower extremity and pelvic mobility while developing a strong inner and outer core. Since disc issues tend to reoccur, it's critical that you make the appropriate life style changes (specifically, when addressing chronic sitting and poor posture issues). Maintain a long term lumbar strengthening program for prevention.

STENOSIS

Stenosis of the spine refers to a narrowing of the space where the nerves exit the spine and go into the extremities. This typically occurs due to arthritis and boney formation along the foraminal opening where the nerve exits. Pain from stenosis can generally be managed conservatively, but if the pain is severe or if you are experiencing "red flag" symptoms, such as a loss of sensation or loss of bowel/bladder control (as in **Initial Treatment**), then lumbar surgery may need to be performed.

As with all cases of spinal pain, maintaining a strong inner and outer core and posterior chain is critical. However, pain from stenosis can be unique as it often responds well to flexion biased exercises. (Typically, lumbar extension seems to work better for most other types of pain.) If you follow the principle of directional preference, those suffering from stenosis usually discover that symptoms resolve with flexion biased movements. This will be an important factor to remember as stenosis is a long term problem that will not heal without surgical intervention. The symptoms that tend to come and go. As you experience pain and symptoms, return to the particular exercises that reduce or eliminate that pain, and then continue back to your exercise program.

DEGENERATIVE DISC DISEASE (DDD) – ARTHRITIS

Degenerative Disc Disease (DDD), a junk term used by many physicians and radiologists, is a common diagnosis. It's probably the worst term ever used in medicine because it sounds scary and is misleading. It's very non-specific. DDD is not a disease and will not lead to death.

I tend to look at DDD as nothing more that arthritis in the spine and/or vertebrae. Many people use this term to describe the normal changes that occur in the spinal discs. Even without injury, the discs over time will lose joint spacing and height. This will be accelerated in cases of injury such as disc herniation, instability or some other traumatic event. DDD can lead to other conditions, such as spinal stenosis, but in general, this term doesn't mean much. Although often diagnosed, it may or may be related to the pain you are experiencing.

My advice is to keep it in the back of your mind that your spine is showing signs of aging and wear and tear. Use that as motivation to perform the daily exercises demonstrated in the **Low Back Pain (LBP) – Rehabilitation Guide**.

Exercise and a healthy lifestyle are the keys to maintaining a healthy spine long term. Avoid activities that cause pain. Modify the activities as needed. Continue to work on maximizing strength in the spine and mobility in the pelvis and spine.

PRIOR SURGERIES

There are many different types of spinal surgeries performed. Some are simpler, such as a discectomy or a laminectomy, and some are more complicated like a lumbar fusion. If you have had lumbar surgery, then you need to be aware of the exact surgery, when it was performed, and why.

Regardless of the type of surgery performed, some form of exercise needs to be performed long term. A focus on inner and outer core strength as well as proper posterior chain strength is critical.

Depending on the type of surgery and where you are in the recovery process, certain exercises may need to be modified in the short term or possibly long term (in the case of more severe and involved surgery). If you follow the principle of directional preference along with the advice of your physician and physical therapist, then participation in exercise and activity will be a critical component to long term maintenance. The key is to insure safety for the long term.

A specific diagnosis for your lumbar pain doesn't mean that you can't exercise or participate in your favorite activity again. It only means that you have a name for your pain. Depending on the condition, get your physician's clearance prior to participating in high level activities. Exercise and activity should be an integral component to your treatment. Follow the concept of peripheralization and centralization. Monitor for worsening symptoms.

If you are experiencing ongoing symptoms, ask for help! I would avoid any practitioner that wants to utilize a passive approach over any length of time. The body is designed to move. Movement and exercise are integral to your long term management. Depending on your diagnosis and/or injury, certain movements and activities may need to be modified. Please consult with your physical therapist.

LOW BACK PAIN (LBP)
LONG TERM TREATMENT AND MANAGEMENT

The good news is that low back pain (LBP) shouldn't prevent you from exercising. Once you have recovered from the initial acute phase, then a return to exercise is an important component to long term management.

Initially as part of a long term strategy, address the patterns that led to or increased your risk of developing LBP. This may also include lifestyle choices such as smoking. In almost all cases, this will include addressing chronically poor posture while sitting and standing; excessive sitting; and flexion activities.

As part of your management strategy, weekly targeted exercise to maintain and improve lumbar extensor and posterior chain strength will be critical. **Your baseline minimum should be to perform at least 10 minutes a week of focused lumbar paraspinal muscle strengthening.** Even 10 minutes a week has been shown to be an effective method to control and prevent low back pain. I recommend that you perform the **Core Strengthening Exercises – Lumbar Extensors** as part of your daily prevention strategy (working toward 10 minutes per day).

LOW BACK PAIN (LBP) MANAGEMENT TIPS AND TECHNIQUES

- You must address the factors that led to the episode of LBP. Eliminate as many risk factors as you can. Address chronically poor posture while sitting and standing; excessive sitting; and flexion activities.

- Re-read the list of potential **Risk Factors for Low Back Pain (LBP),** and then eliminate as many of them as you can.

- Be a zealot about implementing the recommended prevention strategies. Never skip or rush the process.

- In case you missed it, don't skip your warm up!

- Initiate a daily (or nearly daily) lumbar and pelvic range of motion and lumbar strengthening protocol.

- Try to avoid lumbar flexion (particularly, at near end of range flexion and especially, under load).

- Try to avoid lumbar rotation (particularly, under load or in combination with flexion).

- Avoid uncontrolled eccentric movements. Examples include: moving down into a squat; returning down after a dead lift; and running out of control downhill.

For CrossFitters, an example of an uncontrolled eccentric descent is the downward motion after performing a box jump. Try to land with soft knees to absorb the landing pressures through the legs so that you can immediately jump again in order to make the exercise more plyometric in nature. This would hold true for any time that you are coming back down from a jump. Allow the legs to absorb more force and reduce the strain on the lumbar spine. **Eccentric movements always need to be performed under control.**

- Avoid lifting or performing any exercise beyond your technical capability or capacity. This also means not to perform an exercise under load that you don't have the adequate range of motion to actually perform the movement.

- Always use perfect form and technique. On every lift, every time. Be especially vigilant as you fatigue or if you are in a higher volume or high intensity stage of your training plan.

- When performed correctly, every exercise should be a "core" exercise. Fully engage your core stabilizing muscles during any movement and activity.

- Address any asymmetry related issues. This may be addressing that weak knee you injured 5 years ago or addressing a leg length discrepancy. Keep the body as symmetrical as possible to avoid unnecessary and potentially, dangerous compensation patterns. Spend time spot training these weak areas. It will be worth the effort!

- Develop a thorough recovery protocol and implement it! Your recovery should be as thought out and programmed as your training. Injury prevention should be a factor that is thought about beforehand, so that you can implement a prevention strategy. (Particularly, if you have experienced a lumbar injury previously.)

Statistically, most of us will suffer from an episode of low back pain (LBP). Once we have experienced it, we are forever at a higher risk of a subsequent episode. If you proactively treat the initial or next episode of pain, you can significantly reduce your risk of developing another one. Do whatever you can to eliminate your risk factors for developing LBP. Implement the **Low Back Pain (LBP) Prevention Strategies** as well as these management tips and techniques.

Whether you are a weightlifter, CrossFitter, runner, sport enthusiast, weekend warrior or stay at home parent, your goal should be to have the strongest, most developed lumbar extensor, posterior chain, and core musculature possible along with adequate lower extremity flexibility. Let's get started!

LOW BACK PAIN (LBP) REHABILITATION GUIDE

EXTENSION BIASED STRETCHES FOR LOW BACK PAIN

The following extension biased exercises can be helpful for relieving pain and improving lumbar mobility. They also promote movement throughout the lumbar spine including the discs. Such movement allows for improved nutrient exchange which can assist the healing process.

Most of the time, the best treatment course will be with an extension biased program, but not always. If you attempt an extension biased program and the pain worsens, then try the flexion biased movements.

The rule of thumb for movement: **If the pain worsens by spreading peripherally down the buttock and into the leg and/or foot, then the condition is worsening. We must stop that activity. If the pain centralizes and returns back toward the spine (even if the pain worsens slightly), then keep moving as the condition is actually improving.** For a thorough discussion and an excellent treatment resource, please refer to ***Treat Your Own Back*** by Robin A. McKenzie.

Press-ups

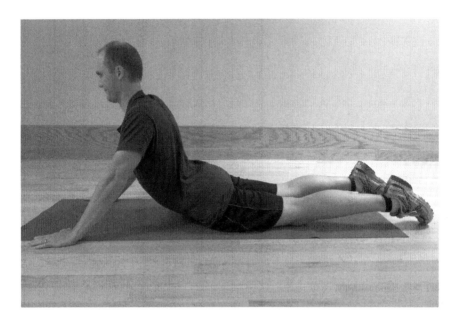

» Perform press-ups before and after running or exercise as part of a thorough warm up and cool down. I also recommend performing press-ups as needed for LBP prevention frequently throughout the day. Lie on your stomach and perform 10 to 20 press-ups. Move slow and easy, but work your way up to full motion.

» Perform 2 sets of 10-20 repetitions, 5-10 times per day.

Standing Back Extension

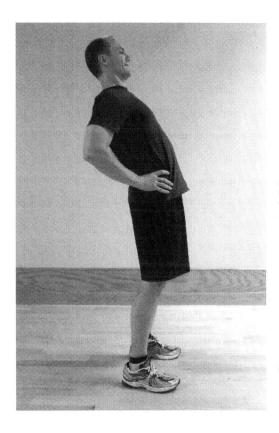

» After sitting, stand up, and perform standing back extensions. I encourage performing at least 10 repetitions each time you stand. You can lean your buttock against a counter top and extend backwards for an added stretch.

» Perform at least 10 repetitions, multiple times per day.

FLEXION BIASED STRETCHES FOR LOW BACK PAIN

Knee to Chest

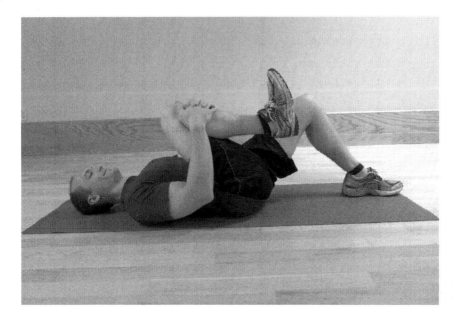

» Pull your knee toward your chest until you feel a stretch in your buttock area. Your other leg can be bent (as shown) or straight.

» Hold for 30 seconds, and 3 repetitions per side.

Double Knee to Chest

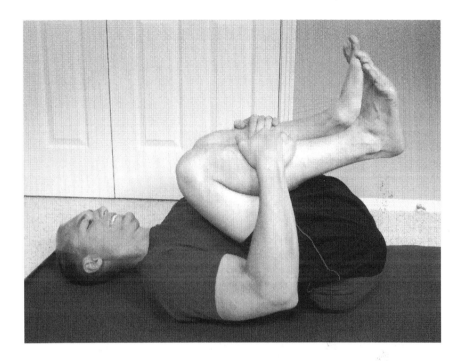

» Pull both knees toward your chest until you feel a stretch in your buttock area. Be sure to keep your head on the ground. Only initiate this exercise if you are able to perform a single knee to chest without peripheralization of symptoms. *These are to be performed only if the directional preference is towards flexion.*

» Hold for 1-2 seconds, perform 10-20 repetitions.

Seated Flexion

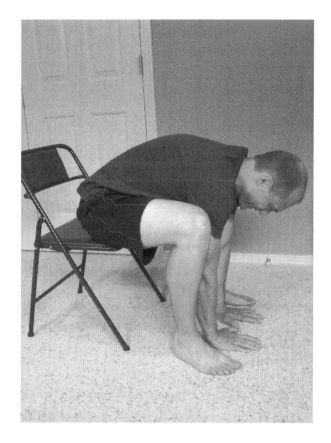

» Gently lean forward and try to touch your hands to the floor. Only initiate this exercise if you are able to perform the double knee to chest without peripheralization of symptoms. *This exercise is to only be performed only if the directional preference is towards flexion.*

» Hold for 1-2 seconds, perform 10-20 repetitions.

LEG AND PELVIC STRETCHES FOR LOW BACK PAIN

As part of any lumbar prevention and treatment protocol, lower extremity and pelvic mobility should be addressed. The legs, pelvis, and low back all work together. Tightness in the legs and pelvis will affect the low back just as poor lumbar mobility will affect the rest of the posterior chain all the way down to the feet. Adequate lower extremity and pelvic mobility takes pressure off of the lumbar spine and promotes symmetry with movement. Symmetry with movement is one way to help to prevent injury.

Hip Flexor – Stretch 1

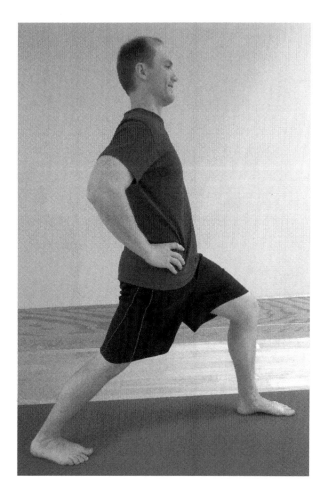

» Stand with good posture with your back leg straight. Keep your back heel on the ground with your toes pointed straight ahead. Flex your front knee until you feel a stretch in the front of your hip. You will also likely feel a stretch in the back of your calf.

» You should feel a mild to moderate stretching sensation and no increase in pain.

» Hold for 30 seconds, and 3 repetitions per side.

Hip Flexor - Stretch 2

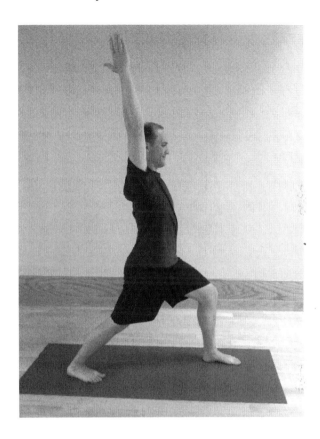

» Stand with good posture with your back leg straight. Keep your back heel on the ground with your toes pointed straight ahead. Flex your front knee until you feel a stretch in the front of your hip. You will also likely feel a stretch in the back of your calf.

» Raise the same arm as your back leg to increase the stretch in the hip flexor area.

» You should feel a mild to moderate stretching sensation and no increase in pain.

» Hold for 30 seconds, and 3 repetitions per side.

Hamstring Stretch in Doorway

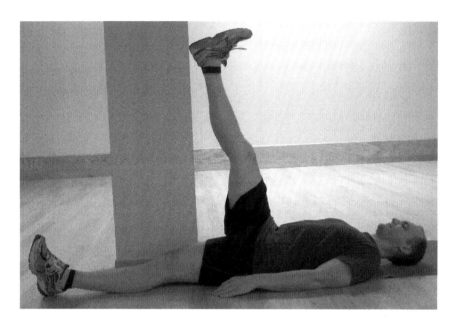

» Find a doorway and place one leg on the frame and stretch the opposite leg through the doorway. Try to keep your back with a neutral arch. As your hamstring relaxes, slowly move closer to the wall or doorframe.

» Hold for at least 1 minute per side, and preferably 2 repetitions per side.

Figure 4 Stretch

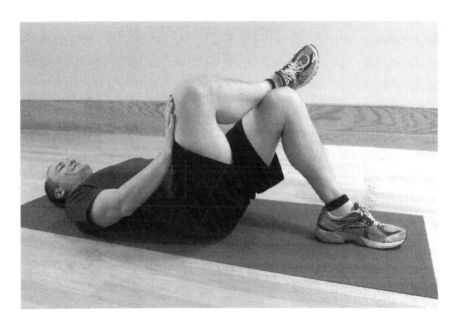

» Cross one leg over the other into a figure 4 position. Push your
   leg away from your head (as shown).

» Hold for 30 seconds, and 3 repetitions per side.

Piriformis Muscle Stretch

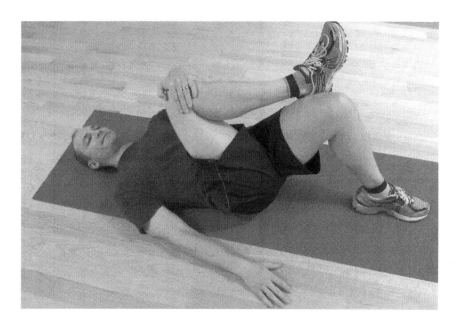

» Cross one leg over the other into a figure 4 position. Hold the opposite leg (while maintaining the figure 4 position) and pull your bent leg toward your chest until you feel a stretch in your buttock area.

» Hold for 30 seconds, and 3 repetitions per side.

Pigeon Stretch

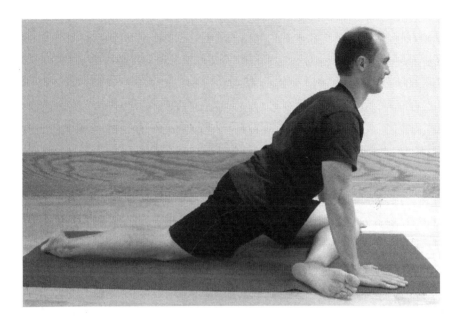

» **This advanced stretch should only be performed in a pain free range for your back.** Keep your front leg with the knee at 90 degrees and straight out in front with your back leg straight behind you. Lean forward as far as you can until you feel a stretch in your buttock. Do not twist your body.

» Hold for 30 seconds, and 3 repetitions per side.

CORE STRENGTHENING EXERCISES – LUMBAR EXTENSORS

Adequate lumbar extension strength is critical to the prevention and treatment of low back pain (LBP). There are many muscle groups in the lumbar spine that assist with extension. Some primarily move the spine while others are more focused on guiding the movement of the spine. These smaller muscles prevent excessive shearing forces from occurring during movement and exercise. In the presence of pain, these small muscles will reflexively turn off. Therefore, your back will be vulnerable to repeated injury.

Without specific training, these muscles will not regain their prior level of function. They will turn off with every associated bout of low back pain. With each occurrence of LBP, you have to specifically work these muscles in order for them to function properly again. The key is to frequently utilize these muscles and to focus on their strength both during an episode of LBP and as part of a prevention strategy.

The exercises below are listed easiest to hardest. **Start with the superman and bridging exercise progression at the same time.** When you are able to, progress from the easier exercises (involving just the arm raise or just a leg raise) onto the more advanced exercises. If you have a repeat bout of pain, start over with your progression. Once you can easily (and nearly pain free) perform an exercise for the recommended sets and repetitions, then it's time to progress to the next exercise.

As you progress, you may want to add 1set of 10-15 repetitions (completing 30 repetitions total). Add weight to increase the resistance when performing ball extensions. Typically, 5-25 lbs. is adequate.

As part of your prevention protocol, perform the following exercises indefinitely: ball bridge with leg raise; ball extension; and the plank. Combine these with press-ups and the **Leg and Pelvic Stretches for Low Back Pain**.

Utilize the Roman chair to perform extensions for repetitions and also for time. If available in your area, utilize a lumbar extension machine known as the **Lumbar MedX**. It's probably the single best lumbar extensor exercise. Straight leg dead lifts and dead lifts should also be part of a long term maintenance program.

Superman Exercise – Starting Position

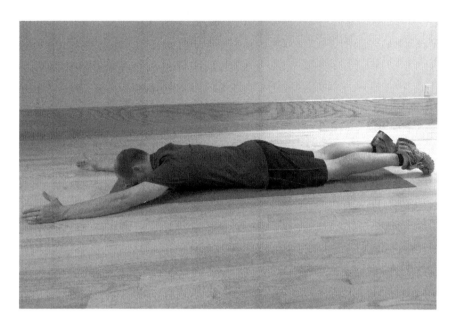

» Lie on the ground with your arms stretched out in a "V" position. Support your head with a small rolled up towel to maintain a neutral spine, and keep your chin slightly tucked.

» You can lie on the floor or a bed. If you are on a bed, you may need a pillow under your stomach for extra support and comfort.

Superman Exercise - Legs

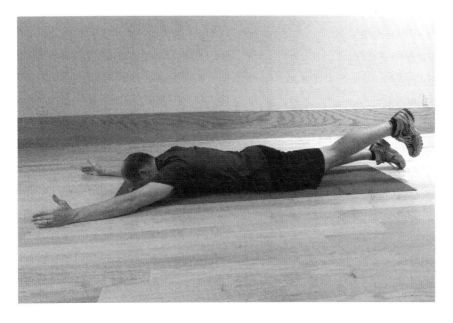

» Raise one leg at a time while being sure to keep your abdominal muscles active. Don't arch your back. Raise your leg up 4-6 inches if you can. If you start to twist in the trunk or low back, then stop. Only raise the leg as far as you can without twisting.

» Perform 2 sets of 10 repetitions, 1-2 times per day.

Superman Exercise – Arms and Legs (Opposite)

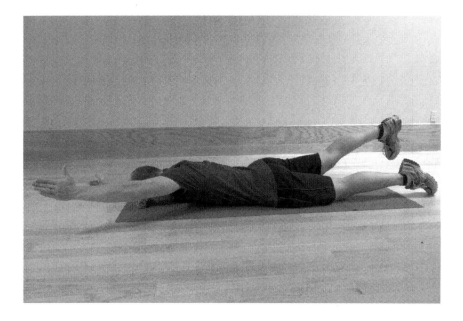

» Raise your opposite arm and leg. Be sure to keep your abdominal muscles active. Don't arch your back. Raise your leg up 4-6 inches if you can. If you start to twist in the trunk or low back, then stop. Only raise the leg as far as you can without twisting. Be sure to keep your chin slightly tucked and in a neutral position. Keep your shoulder blades back and down. Don't shrug.

» Perform 2 sets of 10 repetitions, 1-2 times per day.

Superman Exercise – Arms and Legs (Same Time)

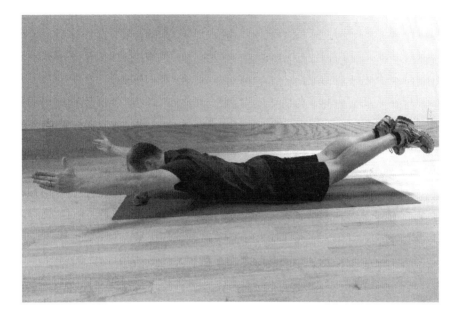

»   Raise your arms and legs. Be sure to keep your abdominal muscles active. Don't over arch your back. Raise your legs up 4-6 inches if you can. As your head elevates, be sure to keep your chin slightly tucked and in a neutral position. Keep your shoulder blades back and down.

»   Perform 1 set of 5 repetitions. Hold each repetition for 30 seconds, 1-2 times per day.

Bridge Exercise – Starting Position

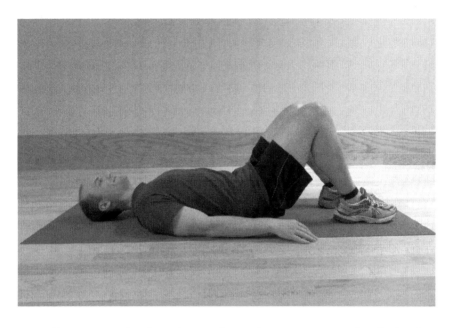

» Lie on your back with your knees bent to prepare for the bridge exercise.

Bridge Exercise

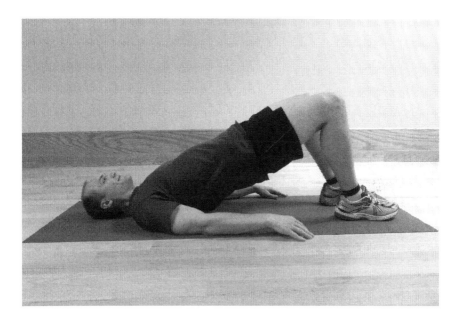

» Keep your pelvis level as you lift your hips/pelvis and buttocks into the air. Pause, and then return back down to the ground. Do not let your pelvis wobble as you move up and down. Add a weight to your pelvis to increase the difficulty level.

» Perform 2 sets of 15 repetitions, 1-2 times per day.

Bridge with March Exercise

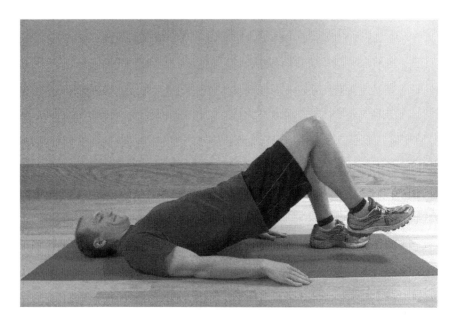

» Keep your pelvis level as you lift your hips/pelvis and buttocks into the air. Alternate marching your feet. Pause, and then return back down to the ground. Do not let your pelvis wobble as you move up and down.

» Perform 2 sets of 10 repetitions, 1-2 times per day.

Ball Bridge Exercise

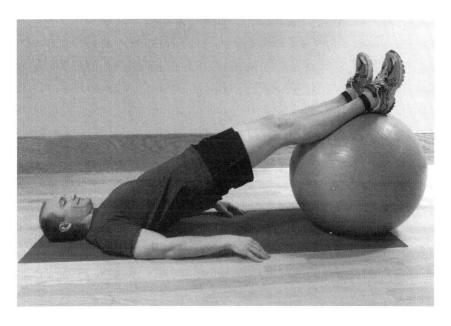

» Keep your pelvis level as you lift your hips/pelvis and buttocks into the air. Pause, and then return back down to the ground. Do not let your pelvis wobble as you move up and down.

» Perform 2 sets of 15 repetitions, 1-2 times per day.

Ball Bridge with Leg Raise Exercise

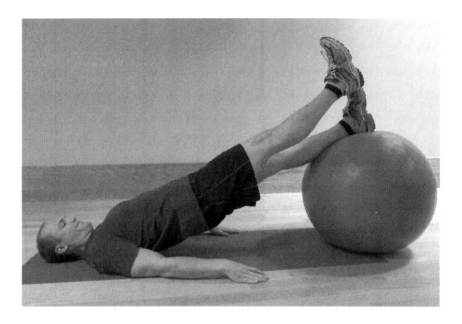

» Keep your pelvis level as you lift your hips/pelvis and buttocks into the air. Pause, raise one leg about 8 inches, then return it to the ball and raise the other. Move slowly. If you are strong enough, then perform all 10 repetitions before lowering your buttock back down to the ground. Do not let your pelvis wobble as you move up and down or when lifting your legs.

» Perform 2 sets of 10 repetitions, 1-2 times per day.

Ball Extension – Starting Position

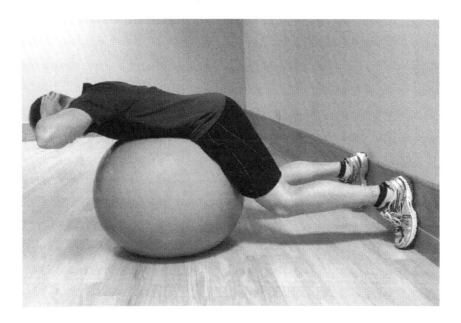

» Position your feet against a wall to assist you with your balance. Your legs stay straight. Keep your chin down in a neutral position and your hands crossed behind your head. You can cross your arms over your chest to make it easier. For more of a challenge, stretch both of your arms into the "V" position (as shown in the superman exercise) or add a weight across the chest.

Ball Extension

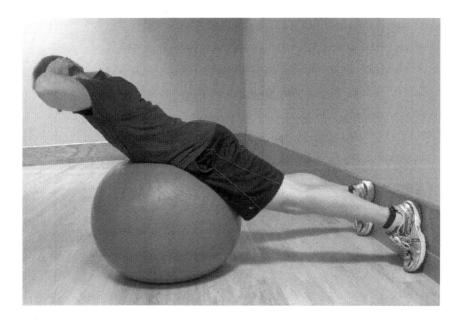

» From your starting position, slowly raise your upper body until you have a slight arch in your back. Keep the movement pain free. To increase the difficulty, add weight either behind your head or hold it across your chest. Start with 5 lbs. and progress up to 15-20 lbs. as you are able.

» Perform 2 sets of 20 repetitions, 1-2 times per day.

Plank Exercise

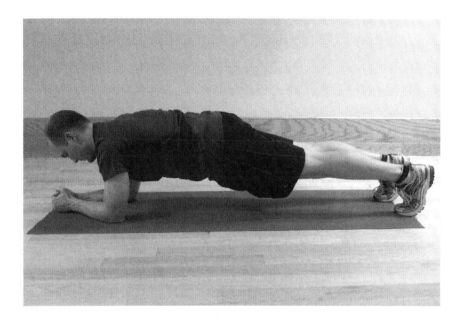

» Keep your chin tucked down so you're looking straight into the ground. Your thighs, buttocks, stomach and back muscles are all engaged. Your elbows should be directly under your shoulders. Keep your body straight, do not tilt.

» Perform 2 sets of 30-60 seconds, once per day.

Side Plank Exercise

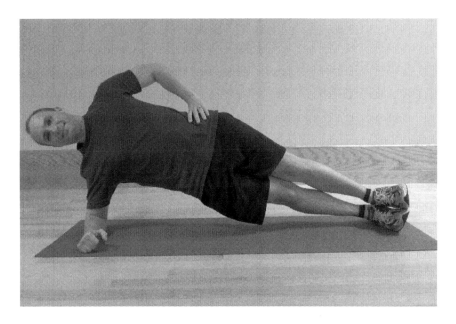

> » Keep your pelvis and shoulders in alignment. Elbow directly under the shoulder. Feet together, pelvis lifted, and your core muscles engaged. Do not tilt, twist or roll backward. For increased difficulty, straighten your top arm upward.

> » Perform 2 sets of 30-60 seconds, once per day.

Roman Chair (Extensions) – Starting Position

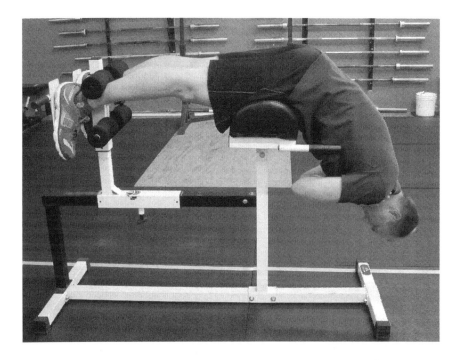

» Position the Roman Chair so that your feet are against the foot rests and your pelvis is held in place by the pad. You should still be able to freely move in your spine. Cross your arms over your chest (as shown) or head or extend them in a superman or "V" position.

Roman Chair (Extensions) - Ending Position

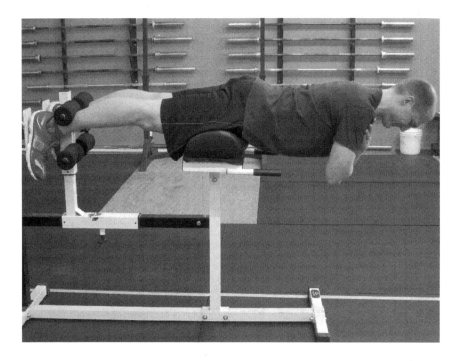

» Extend your torso and focus on activating the back extensor muscles. Extend upright until your body is at least parallel to the ground or in a slight amount of hyper extension. Move slowly. Focus on controlling the movement. You may add weight to add difficulty as long as the movements remain slow and controlled.

» Perform 3 sets of 15 repetitions once per day.

Roman Chair (Static Holds)

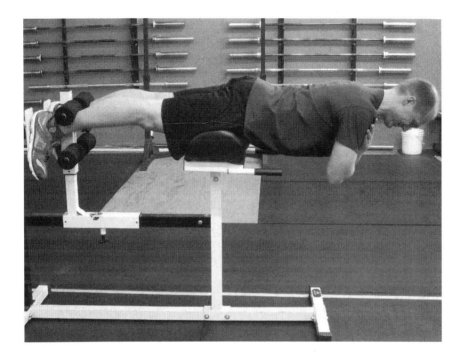

» Position the Roman Chair so that your feet are against the foot rests and your pelvis is held in place by the pad. You should still be able to freely move in your spine. Cross your arms over your chest (as shown) or head or extend them in a superman or "V" position.

» Begin with 3 sets of 30-60 second holds once per day. Hold the position for time. Work up to a longer hold.

CORE STRENGTHENING AND FULL BODY EXERCISES – EMPHASIS ON LUMBAR EXTENSORS

As you progress with your core specific exercises, you will also want to progress back into specific full body strength training exercises that also cause high activation of the core and lumbar extensor muscles. These exercises specifically activate the posterior chain. Progress slowly. There shouldn't be any increase in pain from these exercises. Be sure to follow the rule of thumb for movement.

Once you can perform these exercises at a moderate weight, it will be time to progress into all of your activities that you were participating in prior to injury or an episode of LBP. Continue to progress your core and lumbar extensor strength. Include these core and lumbar extensor strengthening exercises as part of your long term training.

Good Mornings – Starting Position

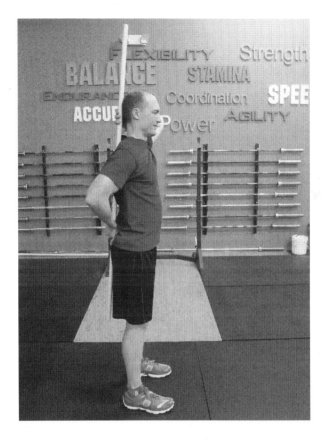

» Use a wooden dowel or PVC pipe. There should be 3 points of contact: back of the head, upper back, and buttock/sacral area. Hold the pole tight against these areas. This will teach you how to bend at the hips while not flexing the lumbar spine. This is an important concept as you add weights to this exercise or perform a straight leg dead lift. Power generation needs to come from the buttocks and hamstrings and not just the lumbar extensors. This exercise will help you learn how to control each muscle group independent of the other.

Good Mornings – Flexed Position

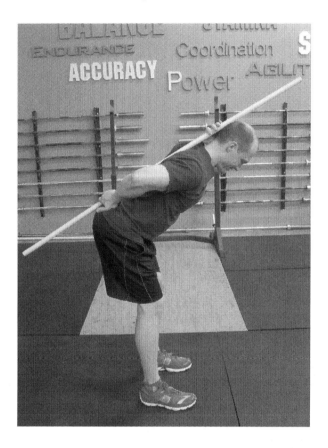

» The initial 3 points of contact: back of the head, upper back, and buttock/sacral area should still be against the pole. The knees remain straight, but not locked into position. Flex from the hips as far as you can until you can no longer maintain the proper form. Then return to standing while maintaining contact with the pole. Keep the inner core muscles active throughout the movement.

» Perform 2 sets of 15 repetitions once per day.

Good Mornings with Weight – Starting Position

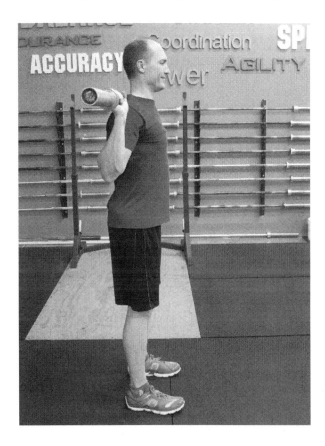

» Once you have mastered the movement pattern without weight, you can attempt to add weight. Start light and work your way up. There shouldn't be any increase in your low back pain during the movement. The spine must maintain its natural lumbar curve. The knees remain straight, but not locked into position. Flex from the hips as far as you can until you can no longer maintain the proper form.

Good Mornings with Weight – Ending Position

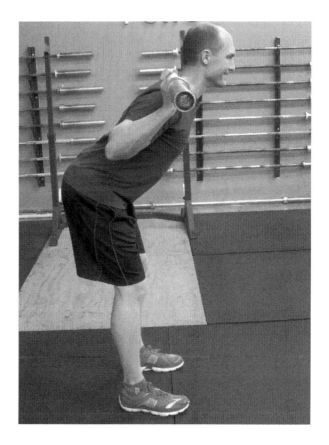

» Flex from the hips. The spine must maintain its natural lumbar curve. The knees remain straight, but not locked into position. As you flex from the hips go as far as you can until you can no longer maintain the proper form. Then return to standing. Keep the inner core muscles active throughout the movement.

» Perform 2 sets of 15 repetitions once per day.

Straight Leg Dead Lifts – Starting Position

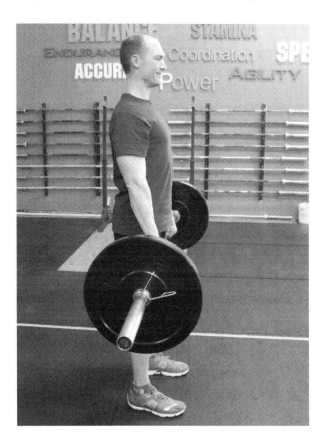

» This exercise will teach you how to bend at the hips while not flexing the lumbar spine. This exercise is designed to work on posterior chain strength (particularly, the glutes/buttocks and hamstrings). The role of the lumbar extensors should be to stabilize during the movement. It's critical that you actively engage the muscles of the inner core and that the lumbar spine maintains its natural lumbar curve. This exercise will help you learn how to control each muscle group independent of the other.

Straight Leg Dead Lifts – Ending Position

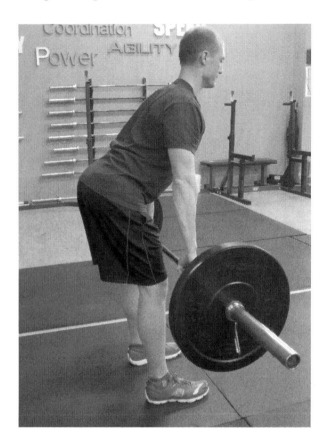

» Flex from the hips. The spine must maintain its natural lumbar curve. The knees remain straight, but not locked into position. As you flex from the hips, move as far as you can until you can no longer maintain the proper form. Then return to standing. Keep the inner core muscles active throughout the movement.

» Begin with a light weight. Perform 2 sets of 15 repetitions once per day. As you fully recover, perform this exercise as a more strength based protocol. For example, 5 sets of 5 repetitions.

Dead Lifts – Starting Position

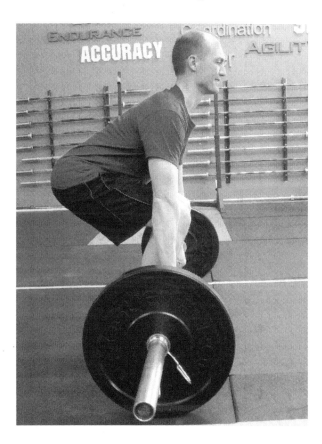

» This exercise is designed to work on posterior chain strength (glutes/buttocks, hamstrings, and back extensors). It's critical that you actively engage the muscles of inner core. Be sure to initiate the movement with the legs, not the spine.

Dead Lifts – Ending Position

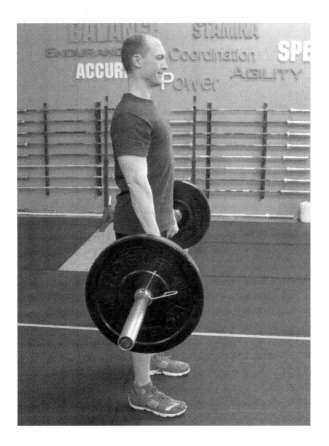

» Be sure to stand all the way up. Initially, you may want to drop the weights versus lowering them back down. The eccentric phase can be the most difficult post recovery. Eventually, it will be critical to control both the eccentric and concentric phases of motion.

» Begin with a light weight. Perform 2 sets of 15 repetitions once per day. As you fully recover, perform this exercise as a more strength based protocol. For example, 5 sets of 5 repetitions.

Single Leg Dead Lifts

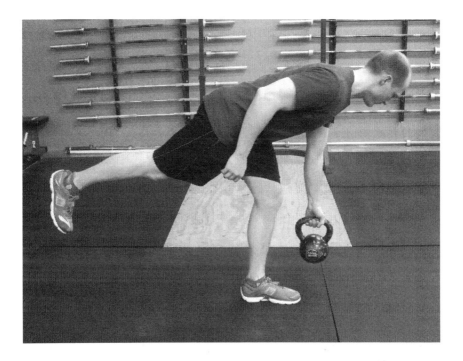

» Start by standing upright. Then slowly bend forward at the hip while keeping the stance leg straight. Keep your spine's natural lumbar curve and keep the pelvis level. Return to standing. Move slowly. Once the technique has been mastered, add resistance (as shown). You can vary the exercise by adding weight to the same side of the stance leg or to the opposite side of the stance leg. Always focus on technique, not weight.

» Perform 2 sets of 15 repetitions each leg once per day.

Focus additional attention and training to the lumbar extensors and muscle of the posterior chain prior to returning to full sport or exercise activities. The descriptions of these exercises are basic. If you (and I highly recommend that you do) participate in weight training as a sport or as a means to improve in your desired sport, then you should invest in learning proper technique and training protocols when utilizing basic and advanced barbell training techniques. I highly recommend that you read Mark Rippetoe's *Starting Strength: Basic Barbell Training*.

LOW BACK PAIN – KINESIOLOGICAL TAPING

There are several different brands of kinesiology style tape. I have had luck using **Kinesio Tape**, **Rock Tape**, **KT Tape**, and **Mummy Tape** brands. There are many other useful taping techniques which utilize different forms of tape. Below are two examples of methods I use to tape for low back pain.

You will need assistance in applying the tape. Cut the strips to length. Remember to cut them a little shorter as the tape will stretch when applied. Be sure to round the corners of the tape prior to applying. This helps to keep it from catching on clothing. The tape is heat activated. This means it gets stickier as it warms up to your body temperature. **Apply the tape at least 30 minutes prior to activity.** The tape can get wet as long as you allow it to dry thoroughly. You could even use a hair dryer if the tape becomes wet.

When applying either of these techniques, first identify the painful area. Slightly lean over when the tape is applied. Be sure that the application of the tape is over the painful area.

"H" TECHNIQUE

Kinesiological Taping for Low Back Pain (LBP)

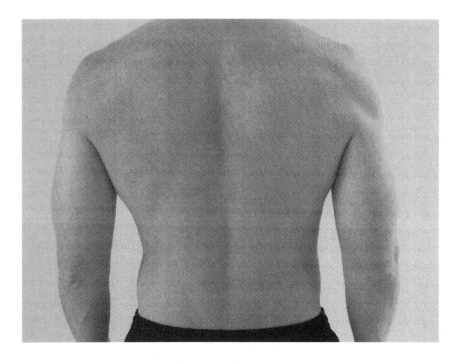

» Identify the painful area and be sure that the application of the tape is over the painful area. You will need assistance in applying the tape. Slightly lean over when applying the tape.

» Cut the strips to length and be sure to round the corners of the tape.

Tape Application for "H" Technique – Stage 1

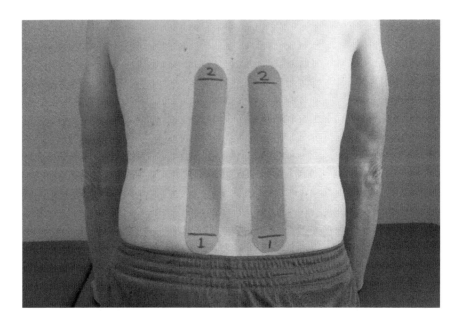

» Remove approximately 1 inch of the backing on the tape. Without stretching it, apply the 1 inch section of tape along the lumbar para spinal muscles (as shown). The middle portion of the tape should contain 50-75% stretch while the ends have no stretch. Be sure to cut the strips long enough to be several inches past the painful area in both directions.

"H" Technique – Stage 2

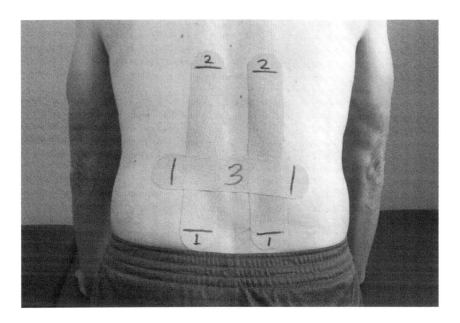

» Apply the third strip of the tape over the painful area. Remove approximately 1 inch of the backing on the tape and apply without stretch. Then apply a 50-75% stretch horizontally across the spine with the other end finishing with the last 1 inch without a stretch.

» If you feel additional horizontal strips are needed, then add them now. Make sure that the tape is securely fashioned to your skin. You may want to rub it back and forth briskly to heat up the tape, which will increase its stickiness.

"H" Technique – Completed

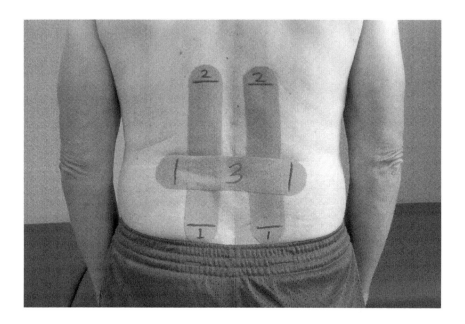

» Stand up. This is how the application should look upon completion.

» **The tape should be applied at least 30 minutes prior to exercise.**

STAR TECHNIQUE

Kinesiological Taping for Low Back Pain (LBP) – Star Technique

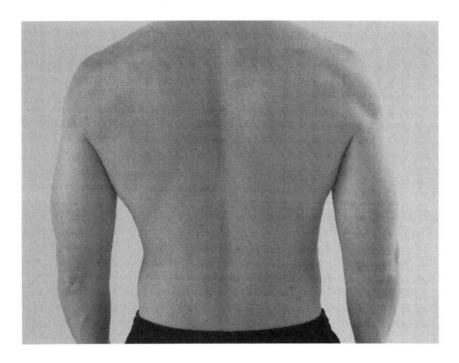

» Identify the painful area and be sure that the application of the tape is over the painful area. You will need assistance in applying the tape. Slightly lean over when applying the tape.

» Cut the strips to length and be sure to round the corners of the tape.

Tape Application for Star Technique – Stage 1

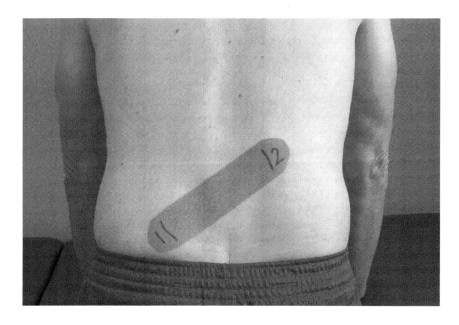

» Start with the diagonal pieces. In Stage 3, you will finish with the horizontal piece.

» Remove approximately 1 inch of the backing on the tape. Without stretching it, apply the 1 inch section of tape starting at one side of the spine crossing over to the other side. Apply 50-75% stretch from one side of the spine when crossing over to the other side. Finish with the last 1 inch without a stretch.

Star Technique – Stage 2

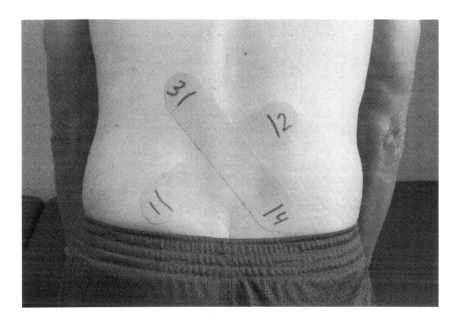

» Remove approximately 1 inch of the backing on the tape for the second strip. Without stretching it, apply the 1 inch section of tape starting at the other side of the spine crossing over (as shown). Apply 50-75% stretch from one side of the spine when crossing over to the other side. Finish with the last 1 inch without a stretch.

Star Technique – Stage 3

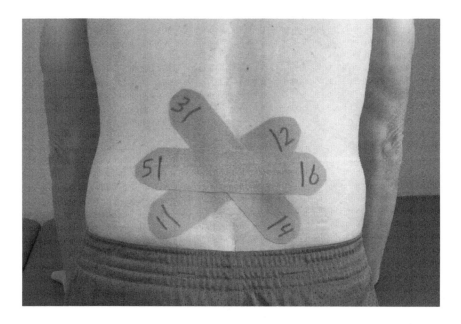

» Remove approximately 1 inch of the backing on the tape, and apply the final strip without stretch. Then apply a 50-75% stretch horizontally across the spine with the other end finishing with the last 1 inch without a stretch. The painful area should be in the middle of the "star".

» If you feel additional strips are needed, then add them now. Make sure that the tape is securely fashioned to your skin. You may want to rub it back and forth briskly to heat up the tape, which will increase its stickiness.

Star Technique – Completed

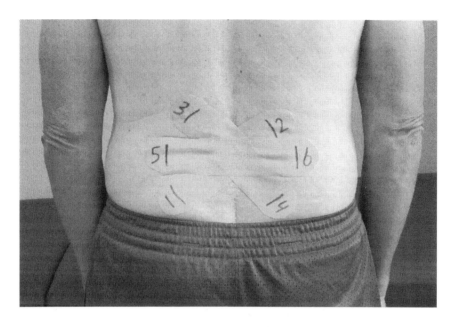

» Stand up. This is how the application should look upon completion.

» **The tape should be applied at least 30 minutes prior to exercise.**

SKIN CARE WITH TAPING

Wearing

- **Round the edges prior to application.**

  Rounding the corners helps to insure that the edges do not catch on clothing and come off prematurely.

- **Prepare the skin initially.**

  Be sure that the skin is clean and free from dirt, body oils, and lotions. You may want to use a special skin preparation liquid designed to protect the skin. Apply first, and allow it to thoroughly dry before applying the tape. Body hair may need to be removed using scissors or clippers, but I do not recommend shaving the area right before application of the tape as this tends to be irritating to the skin.

- **The tape can be worn for several days.**

  Generally the tape can stay on for 4-5 days. Many people are able to wear the tape for a week or so. This may vary with the area being taped and your individual skin. Discuss this with your physical therapist.

- **Shower with the tape on.**

  The tape is water resistant and water proof. You may shower and swim with the tape on. Once out of the water, pat the tape dry or you could even use a hair dryer.

Removal

- **Remove the tape in the direction of hair growth.**

  If you remove the tape in the opposite direction, it gives a "waxing" type of effect and may pull the hair out.

- **Pull your skin off of the tape.**

  Do not pull the tape off of your skin like a Band-Aid. Peel the tape back on itself and work the skin off of the tape as you peel the tape. Pulling away from the body at a 90 degree angle can pull off layers of skin, which causes redness and irritation.

- **Moisturize the skin.**

  Apply a light moisturizer to the skin as you normally would in your daily care.

RESOURCE GUIDE

⅃PHYSICALTHERAPYADVISOR
Empowering You to Reach Your Optimal Health!

NOTE: Throughout this rehabilitation guide, I reference books, exercise equipment, products, supplements, topical agents, and web sites that I personally use and recommend to my family, friends, clients, and patients (for use in the clinical setting). For your reference and convenience, these resources are listed at: **www.thephysicaltherapyadvisor.com/resource-guide/**

Some of the links are "affiliate links." This means if you click on the link and purchase the item, I will receive an affiliate commission **at no extra cost to you**. I recommend them because they are helpful and useful, not because of the small commission I make if you decide to buy something.

BOOKS

- *Starting Strength: Basic Barbell Training* by Mark Rippetoe
- *Treat Your Own Back* by Robin A. McKenzie

EXERCISE EQUIPMENT

- Lumbar MedX

PRODUCTS

- Foam Roller
- Kinesio Tape
- KT Tape
- McKenzie Lumbar Roll
- Mummy Tape
- Rock Tape

SUPPLEMENTS

- CapraColostrum by Mt. Capra
- CapraFlex by Mt. Capra
- Mag Glycinate
- Sherpa Pink Gourmet Himalayan Salt
- Thorne Research Magnesium Citrate
- Tissue Rejuvenator by Hammer Nutrition

TOPICAL AGENTS

- Arnica Rub
- Biofreeze

WEB SITES

- The American Physical Therapy Association
- The Physical Therapy Advisor

TREATING LOW BACK PAIN (LBP) DURING EXERCISE AND ATHLETICS VIDEO PACKAGE

www.thephysicaltherapyadvisor.com/store

To help guide you through **Treating Low Back Pain (LBP) during Exercise and Athletics,** I have created a package that you can get access to which includes a 7-part series of instructional videos in which I address the following:

- Low back pain prevention during exercise

- Specific warm ups for exercise and activities

- What really is the "core" and why it matters

- Treatment techniques (including how to apply Kinesiological tape)

- Long term management strategies

Don't miss out on this nearly 60 minutes of actionable advice to prevent and treat LBP as it relates to active individuals, sports, and athletics!

There is also an additional bonus eBook, **Preventing and Treating Overtraining Syndrome**, in which I show you how to recognize the risk factors and symptoms of Overtraining Syndrome (OTS). You'll learn how to utilize prevention strategies to help you develop a personal training strategy that will allow you to push past your limits and prior plateau points in order to reach a state of what is known as overreaching (your body's ability to "supercompensate"). This will speed up your results, so that you can train harder and more effectively than ever before! In addition, learn how to use the foam roller (complete with photos and detailed exercise descriptions) as part of a health optimization program, recovery program, rest day or treatment modality.

Visit the link below to get a 50% off discount on the **Treating Low Back Pain (LBP) during Exercise and Athletics Video Package.** Just enter discount code **LBP50** for half off!

www.thephysicaltherapyadvisor.com/store

MORE SELF-TREATMENT EBOOKS

My goal as a physical therapist and author is to help proactive adults of all ages to understand how to safely self-treat and manage common musculoskeletal, neurological, and mobility related conditions in a timely manner so they can reach their optimal health. With the cost of healthcare on the rise and no sign of that trend improving, it will become even more necessary to have quality self-treatment education available.

Other eBooks you may be interested in:

PREVENTING AND TREATING OVERTRAINING SYNDROME

In this eBook, I show you how to recognize the risk factors and symptoms of Overtraining Syndrome (OTS). You'll learn how to utilize prevention strategies to help you develop a personal training strategy that will allow you to push past your limits and prior plateau points in order to reach a state of what is known as overreaching (your body's ability to "supercompensate"). This will speed up your results, so that you can train harder and more effectively than ever before! In addition, learn how to use the foam roller (complete with photos and detailed exercise descriptions) as part of a health optimization program, recovery program, rest day or treatment modality.

TREATING ANKLE SPRAINS AND STRAINS

In this book, I show you how to effectively self-treat and manage an ankle sprain and/or strain in order to resume your training and normal activities while minimizing the risk of additional damage, injury or re-injury. When you can confidently self-treat, you can limit pain levels, return to activity faster, and prevent reoccurrences. A proper rehabilitation from the initial injury to the full return to sport and/or activity must include a full return to strength, mobility, and balance. I will walk you through the treatment plan on how to rehabilitate your ankle by beginning with the acute phase of rehabilitation through the intermediate (sub-acute) phase of rehabilitation and concluding with a return to full activity and sport. In this step-by-step rehabilitation guide (complete with photos and detailed exercise descriptions), you will discover how to implement prevention and rehabilitation strategies so that you can safely return to activity.

STAY CONNECTED!

THE PHYSICAL THERAPY ADVISOR
Empowering You to Reach Your Optimal Health!

When you subscribe to my e-mail newsletter, I will send you blog posts on how to maximize your health, self-treat those annoying orthopaedic injuries, and gracefully age. To thank you for subscribing, you will automatically gain access to my FREE resources, **10 Minutes per Day Low Back Pain Prevention Guide** and **My Top 8 Stretches to Eliminate Neck, Upper Back, and Shoulder Pain**.

Be sure to join our growing community on Facebook by liking **The Physical Therapy Advisor** where you will receive additional health and lifestyle information!

Please submit your feedback, comments, and/or questions to:

contact@thePhysicalTherapyAdvisor.com

24490420R00089

Made in the USA
Columbia, SC
23 August 2018